Prevention and Screening

Editor

JOANNA L. DROWOS

PRIMARY CARE:
CLINICS IN OFFICE PRACTICE

www.primarycare.theclinics.com

Consulting Editor
JOEL J. HEIDELBAUGH

March 2019 • Volume 46 • Number 1

ELSEVIER

1600 John F. Kennedy Boulevard • Suite 1800 • Philadelphia, Pennsylvania, 19103-2899

http://www.theclinics.com

PRIMARY CARE: CLINICS IN OFFICE PRACTICE Volume 46, Number 1
March 2019 ISSN 0095-4543, ISBN-13: 978-0-323-65527-9

Editor: Jessica McCool
Developmental Editor: Laura Fisher

Primary Care: Clinics in Office Practice (ISSN: 0095-4543) is published quarterly by Elsevier Inc., 360 Park Avenue South, New York, NY 10010-1710. Months of issue are March, June, September, and December. Periodicals postage paid at New York, NY and additional mailing offices. Subscription prices are $246.00 per year (US individuals), $505.00 (US institutions), $100.00 (US students), $303.00 (Canadian individuals), $572.00 (Canadian institutions), $175.00 (Canadian students), $357.00 (international individuals), $572.00 (international institutions), and $175.00 (international students). Foreign air speed delivery is included in all *Clinics* subscription prices. All prices are subject to change without notice. POSTMASTER: Send address changes to *Primary Care: Clinics in Office Practice*, Elsevier Periodicals Customer Service, 11830 Westline Industrial Drive, St. Louis, MO 63146. Customer Service Health Sciences Division, Subscription Customer Service, 3251 Riverport Lane, Maryland Heights, MO 63043. **Customer Service: 1-800-654-2452 (U.S. and Canada); 314-447-8871 (outside U.S. and Canada). Fax: 314-447-8029. E-mail: journalscustomerservice-usa@elsevier.com (for print support); journalsonlinesupport-usa@elsevier.com (for online support).**

Reprints. For copies of 100 or more, of articles in this publication, please contact the Commercial Reprints Department, Elsevier Inc., 360 Park Avenue South, New York, NY 10010-1710. Tel. 212-633-3874; Fax: 212-633-3820; E-mail: reprints@elsevier.com.

Primary Care: Clinics in Office Practice is covered in *MEDLINE/PubMed (Index Medicus)* and *EMBASE/Excerpta Medica, Current Contents/Clinical Medicine, and ISI/BIOMED.*

Contributors

CONSULTING EDITOR

JOEL J. HEIDELBAUGH, MD, FAAFP, FACG
Clinical Professor, Departments of Family Medicine and Urology, University of Michigan Medical School, Ann Arbor, Michigan

EDITOR

JOANNA L. DROWOS, DO, MPH, MBA, CMQ, FACOFP
Associate Professor of Family Medicine, Associate Chair, Integrated Medical Science Department Director, Community and Preventive Medicine Clerkship, Charles E. Schmidt College of Medicine, Florida Atlantic University, Boca Raton, Florida

AUTHORS

BRALIN BEAN, DO
Resident, Residency in Family Medicine, Lakeside Medical Center, Belle Glade, Florida

RUSS BLACKWELDER, MD, MDiv, CMD
Director of Geriatric Education, Assistant Professor, Department of Family Medicine, Medical University of South Carolina, Charleston, South Carolina; Associate Medical Director, The Village at Summerville, Summerville, South Carolina

MATTHEW G. CHECKETTS, DO
Resident Physician, Department of Internal Medicine, Charles E. Schmidt College of Medicine, Florida Atlantic University, Boca Raton, Florida

ALEXANDER CHESSMAN, MD
Professor, Department of Family Medicine, Medical University of South Carolina, Charleston, South Carolina

PHILIP COLLINS, DO
Assistant Professor, Department of Family Medicine, Rowan University School of Osteopathic Medicine, Stratford, New Jersey

PETER EDEMEKONG, MD, MPH
Resident, Residency in General Preventive Medicine and Public Health, Florida Department of Health, Palm Beach County, West Palm Beach, Florida

ZOE FELD, MD
Resident Physician, Department of Obstetrics and Gynecology, University of California, Davis, California

NIKERSON GENEVE, DO
Program Director, Residency in Family Medicine, Lakeside Medical Center, Belle Glade, Florida

JYOTHI GUNTA, MD, MPH
Resident, Residency in General Preventive Medicine and Public Health, Florida Department of Health, Palm Beach County, West Palm Beach, Florida

CHARLES H. HENNEKENS, MD, DrPH
Charles E. Schmidt College of Medicine, Florida Atlantic University, Boca Raton, Florida

ELIZABETH HIDLEBAUGH, MD
Resident Physicians, Department of Internal Medicine, Charles E. Schmidt College of Medicine, Florida Atlantic University, Boca Raton, Florida

ANDREW MANYIN HO, DO
Family Medicine Resident, Family Medicine Residency, Beaumont Health Troy, Sterling Heights, Michigan

ALLISON HOLLEY, MD
Assistant Professor of Integrated Medical Sciences, Division of Medicine, Charles E. Schmidt College of Medicine, Florida Atlantic University, Boca Raton, Florida

VERONICA JORDAN, MD, MS
Faculty, Santa Rosa Family Medicine Residency, Assistant Clinical Professor, University of California, San Francisco, Santa Rosa, California

DANIEL KAIRYS, MD
General Surgeon, Northern Light Maine Coast Hospital, Ellsworth, Maine

MUNEEZA KHAN, MD, FAAFP
Associate Professor, Program Director, Saint Francis Family Medicine Residency, Chair, Department of Family Medicine, The University of Tennessee Health Science Center, Memphis, Tennessee

ALEXANDER KOWALSKI, DO
Assistant Professor, Department of Family Medicine, Rowan University School of Osteopathic Medicine, Stratford, New Jersey

SHOSHANA B. LEVY, MD, MPH
Program Director, Residency in General Preventive Medicine and Public Health, Florida Department of Health, Palm Beach County, West Palm Beach, Florida

LISA C. MARTINEZ, MD
Assistant Professor of Integrated Medical Sciences, Division of Medicine, Charles E. Schmidt College of Medicine, Florida Atlantic University, Boca Raton, Florida

RON MATHEW, DO
Resident, Residency in Family Medicine, Lakeside Medical Center, Belle Glade, Florida

DAVID J. PARK, DO, FAAFP, FACOFP
Professor of Family Medicine, Rocky Vista University College of Osteopathic Medicine–Southern Utah, Ivins, Utah

ERWIN MATTHEW PATALINGHUG, MD
Clinical Faculty, Family Medicine Residency, Beaumont Health Troy, Sterling Heights, Michigan

PARVATHI PERUMAREDDI, DO
Assistant Professor of Biomedical Sciences, Charles E. Schmidt College of Medicine, Florida Atlantic University, Boca Raton, Florida

JOANNA PETRIDES, MBS, PsyD
Assistant Professor, Department of Family Medicine, Rowan University School of Osteopathic Medicine, Stratford, New Jersey

MARC A. PFEFFER, MD, PhD
Division of Cardiovascular Medicine, Harvard Medical School, Brigham and Women's Hospital, Boston, Massachusetts

DONNA PRILL, MD
Senior Associate Director, Clinic Director and Core Faculty, Research Family Medicine Residency, Kansas City, Missouri

TYLER PROVOST, DO
Resident, Residency in Family Medicine, Lakeside Medical Center, Belle Glade, Florida

BERNARDO REYES, MD
Assistant Professor of Geriatric Medicine, Charles E. Schmidt College of Medicine, Florida Atlantic University, Boca Raton, Florida

NICOLE SCHUTTENBERG, BS, MS
Charles E. Schmidt College of Medicine, Florida Atlantic University, Boca Raton, Florida

MANDI SEHGAL, MD
Associate Professor of Geriatric Medicine, Charles E. Schmidt College of Medicine, Florida Atlantic University, Boca Raton, Florida

JENNIFER SEPEDE, DO
Assistant Professor, Department of Family Medicine, Rowan University School of Osteopathic Medicine, Stratford, New Jersey

DAWN SHERLING, MD
Assistant Professor of Integrated Medical Sciences, Division of Medicine, Charles E. Schmidt College of Medicine, Florida Atlantic University, Boca Raton, Florida

RANDI SPERLING, DO, FAAP, FACOP
Assistant Professor of Integrated Medical Science, Division of Pediatrics, Charles E. Schmidt College of Medicine, Florida Atlantic University, Boca Raton, Florida

MARIA STEVENS, MD
Assistant Professor, Department of Humanities, Health, and Society, Herbert Wertheim College of Medicine, Florida International University, Miami, Florida

SARAH E. STUMBAR, MD, MPH
Assistant Professor, Department of Humanities, Health, and Society, Herbert Wertheim College of Medicine, Florida International University, Miami, Florida

NERGESS TAHERI, DO
Resident, Residency in Family Medicine, Lakeside Medical Center, Belle Glade, Florida

MEAGAN VERMEULEN, MD, FAAFP
Assistant Professor, Department of Family Medicine, Rowan University School of Osteopathic Medicine, Stratford, New Jersey

BENJAMIN B. WILDE, DO
Assistant Professor of Family Medicine, Rocky Vista University College of Osteopathic Medicine–Southern Utah, Ivins, Utah

SARAH K. WOOD, MD, FAAP
Senior Associate Dean for Medical Education, Associate Professor of Integrated Medical Science, Division of Pediatrics, Charles E. Schmidt College of Medicine, Florida Atlantic University, Boca Raton, Florida

SRIKALA YEDAVALLY-YELLAYI, DO, MEd
Osteopathic Family Medicine Residency Program Director, Beaumont Health Troy, Family Medicine Clerkship Director, Oakland University William Beaumont School of Medicine, Rochester, Michigan

Contents

Prevention

In primary care, physicians have the opportunity to address preventative causes of morbidity and mortality. Primary care physicians have a distinct opportunity to provide counseling regarding lifestyle changes and disease prevention in a variety of settings, both during the treatment of acute illnesses and with wellness examinations. Questions from patients regarding specific recommendations and interventions are common. In this article, we address barriers to and tools to encourage lifestyle changes in the areas of smoking cessation, weight loss, physical activity, mental health, and substance abuse/misuse.

The increasing burden of cardiovascular disease worldwide, including the United States, underscores the need for the more widespread use of adjunctive drug therapies of proven net benefit in the primary prevention of cardiovascular disease. These include aspirin to reduce mortality from cardiovascular disease, statins to lower LDL-cholesterol levels, appropriate use of multiple antihypertensive drug therapies to lower blood pressure, and aggressive multifactorial management of diabetes. This article reviews randomized evidence to provide guidance to primary care providers regarding the use of adjunctive drug therapies.

Hypertension, among the common conditions encountered in primary care, is known to have a causal link with cardiovascular disease. With new thresholds for diagnosing hypertension, its prevalence is expected to increase. Currently, a high percentage of patients have suboptimal or inadequately controlled blood pressure, thus placing them at risk for cardiovascular disease. Among the best strategies for improved outcomes are inclusion of the patient in decision-making as well as provision of individualized treatment plans.

Screening

leading cause of cancer-related mortality for women in the United States. There are several contradictory recommendations regarding breast cancer screening. Familiarity with these recommendations will allow physicians to counsel their patients and ensure well-informed shared decision making.

Cervical cancer affects the cells lining the cervix, most commonly occurring in the cells of the transformation zone. Screening for cervical cancer looks to detect preinvasive disease, allowing for intervention before invasive disease develops. an assessment of individual risk factors, Selection of screening method depends on patient age, her screening history and results, and resources available. Screening has resulted in well-documented declines in cervical cancer incidence and mortality in the United States. Guidelines continue to evolve as new data emerge. Although cervical cancer prevention strategies include interventions directed toward limiting number of sexual partners, condom use, and reduction in cigarette smoking, vaccination represents the most direct targeted strategy.

This article focuses on programmatic and opportunistic colorectal cancer screening. The pathogenesis and risk factors for colon cancer are discussed. Specific screening tests, screening in high-risk groups, and surveillance recommendations are reviewed. Important considerations for office practice, including improving screening implementation and cost issues, are addressed.

Prostate cancer screening has generated immense interest and controversy in recent years. This article evaluates issues in current prostate cancer pathologic patterns, epidemiology, and screening.

This article discusses sexually transmitted infections (STI) screening and focuses on reportable STIs. This includes gonorrhea, chlamydia, syphilis, and human immunodeficiency virus. Hepatitis B and C, trichomonas, and herpes are covered as well. Recommendations are summarized from the various organizations that produce screening recommendations. These screening recommendations only apply to asymptomatic individuals. Once an individual has symptoms, testing becomes diagnostic. It is important to know the prevalence of STIs within your population. If you work in a population with a high prevalence of a specific disease, you may want to screen regardless of the recommendations.

Update on Osteoporosis

Srikala Yedavally-Yellayi, Andrew Manyin Ho, and Erwin Matthew Patalinghug

Osteoporosis is often a silent disease that reveals itself at the time of a fracture. Assessing risk factors and applying appropriate screening guidelines in the population at risk can potentially decrease the looming high disease burden in the United States. FRAX is a validated tool that can be used to determine 10-year fracture risk to assist in medical decision making. Bone mineral density testing of the hip or spine using DEXA can be used alone or in combination with FRAX to determine patients' risk for fracture and determine if patients are candidates for treatment of osteoporosis.

PRIMARY CARE:
CLINICS IN OFFICE PRACTICE

SERIES OF RELATED INTEREST

Medical Clinics (http://www.medical.theclinics.com)
Physician Assistant Clinics (http://www.physicianassistant.theclinics.com)

THE CLINICS ARE AVAILABLE ONLINE!
Access your subscription at:
www.theclinics.com

Foreword

Prevention into Practice, Practicing Prevention

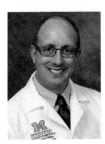

Joel J. Heidelbaugh, MD, FAAFP, FACG
Consulting Editor

Primary care practices are tasked with centering the health care of adults and children, women and men, on the prevention of disease and cancer. Guidelines change, quality metrics loom, and patients continue to occupy a spectrum of interest and engagement relative to prevention and screening. With increasingly complicated agendas during patient encounters coupled with limited time per office visit, meeting the appropriate needs of our patients in teaching disease prevention and in discussing current guidelines while offering unbiased shared decision making remains a formidable challenge.

Over the last two decades, I've been privileged to serve on many guideline panels, spanning gastrointestinal and urological disorders, governed by academic institutions like my current home at the University of Michigan as well as with specialty societies, including the American Gastroenterological Association and the American Urological Association. I've learned a lifetime of education regarding the challenges that beget the development of guidelines, including rigorous literature reviews, statistical analyses, outcomes evaluation, and the impact of the literature, evidence, and final guideline development on patients and populations. What I've realized is that we all want simple answers based upon high-quality evidence, yet such an easy road rarely exists.

This issue of *Primary Care: Clinics in Office Practice* has been uniquely divided into two sections, namely Prevention and Screening. The Prevention section highlights the importance of lifestyle modifications to promote disease prevention, the evidence on aspirin therapy, and strategies to prevent hypertension and diabetes mellitus. This section also highlights current immunization guidelines and strategies for implementation. These articles provide cogent guidance, while presenting advice on how to best educate patients.

Dr David Crawford, a urologist in Colorado and valued colleague of mine, recently stated in a lecture on prostate cancer screening, "*To own the truth, own the data.*" This statement holds special importance to me when I contemplate screening

Prim Care Clin Office Pract 46 (2019) xiii–xiv
https://doi.org/10.1016/j.pop.2018.12.002
0095-4543/19/© 2018 Published by Elsevier Inc.

primarycare.theclinics.com

guidelines, but more specifically on how we need to explain them to patients and offer shared decision making. The Screening section of this issue of *Primary Care: Clinics in Office Practice* covers pertinent pediatric and geriatric screening provisions, while presenting current guidelines on breast, cervical, prostate, and colon cancer screening. The best evidence-based guidelines for these cancers often change, are often conflicted across specialty societies and the US Preventive Services Task Force, and often create confusion in interpretation for primary care providers. Screening guidelines for sexually transmitted infections and osteoporosis are also presented, with greater evidence in favor of screening women than men, yet presenting opportunities for discussion in high-risk populations across both genders.

I would like thank Dr Joanna Drowos and her very knowledgeable colleagues and authors for their outstanding contributions to this important issue of *Primary Care: Clinics in Office Practice.* The topics and guidelines presented herein are of significant importance in our daily primary care practices and will certainly help to guide us in putting prevention into practice, nonetheless practicing prevention.

Joel J. Heidelbaugh, MD, FAAFP, FACG
Departments of Family Medicine and Urology
University of Michigan Medical School
Ann Arbor, MI 48103, USA

Ypsilanti Health Center
200 Arnet, Suite 200
Ypsilanti, MI 48198, USA

E-mail address:
jheidel@umich.edu

Preface

Perspectives on Prevention and Screening

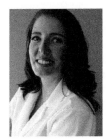

Joanna L. Drowos, DO, MPH, MBA, CMQ, FACOFP
Editor

Each year in the United States, millions of premature deaths result from potentially preventable diseases. These deaths occur from preventable chronic diseases, such as heart disease, cancer, and diabetes, leading to 7 of every 10 deaths and accounting for 75% of our nation's health spending. Preventive care includes health services, such as screenings, physical examinations, and patient counseling, with the goal of preventing illness and disease, or detecting conditions at an early stage when treatment is likely to work best. Preventive services improve health outcomes by either avoiding acquiring the disease in the first place or mitigating the effects of disease by early detection and intervention. Screening programs serve to identify at-risk individuals for disease within a population with the goal of early detection, when treatment works best. Both prevention and screening have the goal of improving the health of populations, and both are essential components of primary care practice. This issue presents and reviews the evidence and best practices supporting preventive and screening services in primary care for diseases that provide the greatest contribution to premature mortality.

Eating healthy, exercising regularly, avoiding tobacco, and receiving preventive services, such as cancer screenings, vaccinations, and preventive visits, are important steps for keeping patients healthy. While these may seem like obvious recommendations to share with patients, the right preventive care at the right stage of life can have a significant impact on future health outcomes and patient well-being. Physicians and health care teams need to do more than merely provide advice; we must inspire our patients to lead healthier lives and become their partner in pursuing evidence-based preventive and screening services. The ultimate goal of prevention is for all Americans to have the opportunity to stay healthy, to avoid or delay the onset of disease, to keep diseases already present from worsening or becoming debilitating, and enabling them to lead productive lives. Preventing disease is also the key to improving our nation's

Prim Care Clin Office Pract 46 (2019) xv–xvii
https://doi.org/10.1016/j.pop.2018.12.001
0095-4543/19/© 2018 Published by Elsevier Inc.

health and controlling rising health care costs. Investing in prevention provides benefits shared by individual patients and communities alike.

While there is increasing evidence supporting preventive and screening activities, statistics also show that most Americans underutilize these services. Utilization rates are even lower for individuals who experience social, economic, or environmental disadvantages. Obstacles to healthy living include lack of access to quality and affordable health care, limited healthy food choices, unsafe living or working environments, and inadequate access to education or employment opportunities. Insurance status also plays a significant role in accessing recommended preventive services; however, even insured individuals may be deterred by cost-sharing requirements, such as deductibles, coinsurance, or copayments. The Affordable Care Act provides many patients access to preventive services, such as mammograms, Pap smears, or flu shots, by waiving coinsurance or deductibles; however, physicians must be aware of all of the potential barriers that may limit patients' pursuit of health-promoting activities. At a minimum, we as physicians should continually seek knowledge of the latest guidelines and recommended practices in the field of prevention. It is our job to know, understand, and help our patients interpret and individualize the appropriate preventive and screening services to pursue.

As such an integral component to so many facets of medical practice and patient health, it is fitting that the topic of Prevention and Screening receives its own special issue of *Primary Care: Clinics in Office Practice*. While prevention and screening are broad topics with continuously evolving evidence, this issue seeks to address the most current and pertinent recommendations in the field. As a physician who is passionate about Public Health and Preventive Medicine, I am both honored and excited to elevate this important subject as guest editor. While in medical school, I concurrently pursued a Master of Public Health degree and began at that early stage of my career to consider the implications of health promotion and disease prevention on the health of populations. This training ignited my passion and started me down a path of improving individual patient and community-wide health outcomes. Further inspiration struck while completing residency training in preventive medicine sponsored by our county health department; when I had the great fortune of meeting Dr Charles Hennekens. His groundbreaking work linking aspirin with improved cardiovascular disease outcomes has saved countless lives and dramatically advanced the field of preventive medicine. Dr Hennekens remains a cherished mentor, colleague, and friend today. My training and dedication to the field led me to a position as Center Director for our county health department's communicable disease clinic, to today, where I inspire medical students to learn prevention and primary care at the Charles E. Schmidt College of Medicine at Florida Atlantic University.

For this special issue, I have assembled a collection of clinicians and educators with broad expertise in prevention and screening topics. Article authors include experts in preventive care for patient populations ranging from pediatric to geriatric, from settings spanning academic, community based, and public health focused. These clinicians and educators continually inspire me to learn more and to update my knowledge as evidence and guidelines evolve. It is humbling to be able to provide the readers of this publication with that same opportunity. Our work is organized into two distinct sections: the first addressing prevention, including primary and secondary activities, and the second offering guidelines for screening of specific preventable diseases among populations.

I am grateful for the opportunity to design and present this special issue on prevention and screening. On behalf of my coauthors, we are pleased to present this resource for your practice. As physicians, it is not only our job to help our patients pursue the appropriate preventive health services but also our privilege to help them lead healthier, more productive lives. Thank you for taking the time to update your knowledge, and for the important work you do each day in improving the lives and health of your patients.

Joanna L. Drowos, DO, MPH, MBA, CMQ, FACOFP
Charles E. Schmidt College of Medicine
Florida Atlantic University
777 Glades Road
Building 71, suite 215
Boca Raton, FL 33431, USA

E-mail address:
JDrowos@health.fau.edu

Prevention

Lifestyle Changes for Disease Prevention

Joanna Petrides, MBS, PsyD*, Philip Collins, DO, Alexander Kowalski, DO, Jennifer Sepede, DO, Meagan Vermeulen, MD, FAAFP

KEYWORDS

- Lifestyle modifications • Smoking cessation • Diet • Physical activity
- Substance abuse • Mental health

KEY POINTS

- Primary care physicians have a distinct opportunity to provide counseling regarding lifestyle changes and disease prevention in a variety of settings.
- The 5 As is one of the models recommended by the US Public Health Service to treat tobacco use and nicotine addiction.
- Lifestyle modifications are the mainstay and cornerstone in treating obesity, and include components such as appropriate meal plans, physical activity, and behavioral interventions for adherence.
- Mental health screening tools are brief approaches to collecting information that can be completed at any time during an office visit.
- Screening for alcohol use disorder and substance abuse should be done systematically and should also address comorbid mental health disorders.

THE PREVENTABLE CAUSES OF MORTALITY

Primary care physicians have a distinct opportunity to provide counseling regarding lifestyle changes at a variety of clinical encounters. Questions regarding specific recommendations and interventions are common. In this article, we address lifestyle changes for preventable mortality such as smoking cessation, weight loss, exercise, mental health, and substance abuse/misuse.

SMOKING CESSATION
Morbidity and Mortality

Tobacco use is one of the top causes of preventable morbidity and mortality globally.[1–3] Tobacco use causes approximately 6 million deaths annually worldwide

Disclosure Statement: The authors have nothing to disclose.
Department of Family Medicine, Rowan University School of Osteopathic Medicine, 42 East Laurel Road, Suite 2100A, Stratford, NJ 08084, USA
* Corresponding author.
E-mail address: petrides@rowan.edu

Prim Care Clin Office Pract 46 (2019) 1–12
https://doi.org/10.1016/j.pop.2018.10.003
0095-4543/19/© 2018 Elsevier Inc. All rights reserved.

primarycare.theclinics.com

including more than 480,000 deaths in the United States alone.[2–5] Second hand smoke results in more than 41,000 deaths per year in the United States related to disease processes such as stroke, lung cancer, heart disease, sudden infant death syndrome, and other respiratory illnesses.[4,5] Based on current trends, it is estimated that tobacco use will lead to 8 million deaths worldwide in 2030.[3] Tobacco use is a risk factor for many diseases such as diabetes, chronic obstructive pulmonary disease, various types of cancers, stroke, heart disease, and other lung diseases such as asthma and pneumonia.[2,4,5] Active smokers ages 25 to 79 years have a death rate 3 times higher than that of people who never smoked. When comparing smokers with people who had never smoked, life expectancy was decreased by at least 10 years for current smokers.[4,6] Within 1 year of quitting, patients decrease their risk of coronary heart disease by 50% and after 4 years of quitting the risk becomes equivalent to a patient who has never smoked. The risk of lung cancer decreases every year that the patient has quit smoking, but the risk will always be higher than someone who never smoked.[1]

Benefits of Smoking Cessation and Strategies for Treatment

In 2015, 68% of adult smokers wanted to attempt smoking cessation and 55.4% of adult smokers attempted to quit smoking at least once in the past year.[4] Research suggests that, compared with persistent smokers, patients who quit smoking between the ages of 25 and 34 years increased their life expectancy by 10 years, whereas smokers who quit smoking between the ages of 35 and 44 years or 45 and 54 years increased their life expectancy by 9 years and 6 years, respectively. Additionally, smoking cessation before the age of 40 years decreased the risk of mortality from smoking-related diseases by 90%.[6]

The US Preventive Services Task Force recommends that physicians ask all adult patients about tobacco use, recommend cessation of tobacco, and provide strategies for smoking cessation such as pharmacotherapy and behavioral interventions.[2] It is also recommended that primary care physicians screen for tobacco use and counsel patients at every visit the likelihood of smoking cessation.[1] The 5 As (**Table 1**) is one of the models recommended by the US Public Health Service to treat tobacco use and nicotine addiction (Ask, Advise, Assess, Assist, and Arrange).[1,2] When used in conjunction with the stages of change model, these tools can be helpful in gauging patient readiness to quit. Once a patient is in the preparation stage, a combination of nicotine replacement, medical therapy, such as bupropion or varenicline, and other support systems, such as quitlines, should be offered to assist with smoking cessation. If a patient is in the precontemplation or contemplation phase, motivational

Table 1 The 5 As	
Ask	Ask each patient at every visit about past and present tobacco use.
Advise	Offer brief counseling about the harms of tobacco use to patients identified as tobacco users.
Assess	Assess the patient's willingness to quit after advice has been given. See **Table 2** for further details.
Assist	Offer smoking cessation strategies to patients willing to quit.
Arrange	Close follow-up such as arranging an appointment 1 wk after the agreed upon quit date.

Data from Refs.[1,2,7]

Table 2	
Stages of change model	
Stage	**Description**
Precontemplation	Patient is not willing to quit within the next 6 mo.
Contemplation	Patient is considering quitting within the next 6 mo, but is not ready to quit right now.
Preparation	Patient is ready to quit in the next 30 d.
Action	Patient has quit smoking successfully for less than 6 mo.
Maintenance	Patient has been without smoking for the last 6 mo.

Data from Okuyemi KS, Nollen NL, Ahluwalia JS. Interventions to facilitate smoking cessation. Am Fam Physician 2006;74(2):262–71; and Larzelere MM, Williams DE. Promoting smoking cessation. Am Fam Physician 2012;85(6):591–8.

interviewing is a great tool the physician can use to help the patient move toward the end goal of smoking cessation.[1,7]

WEIGHT MANAGEMENT
Morbidity and Mortality

The prevalence of obesity continues to increase despite ongoing attention on the matter.[8] It is estimated that 32.7% of US adults aged 20 years and older are overweight, 37.9% are obese, and 7.7% are extremely obese.[9] Obesity is associated with an increased risk of multiple health concerns, including hypertension, type 2 diabetes mellitus, dyslipidemia, obstructive sleep apnea, nonalcoholic fatty liver disease, degenerative joint disease, and some malignancies, thus making obesity a profound concern.[10] Given its association with so many diseases, it is no surprise that obesity is also associated with increased mortality. Compared with normal weight individuals, there is a 50% to 100% increased risk of all-cause mortality with obesity and a diagnosis of overweight accounts for approximately 300,000 deaths per year in the United States.[11] It has also been shown that obesity increases mortality risk among all forms of cancer.[12] As of 2015, the leading causes of death in the United States were heart disease, cancer, unintentional injury, chronic lower respiratory diseases, stroke, Alzheimer's disease, diabetes, influenza and pneumonia, kidney disease, and suicide, all of which obesity can negatively impact and exacerbate.[13]

Determining whether patients are overweight or obese is measured with the body mass index (BMI). The standard for healthy BMI is considered 19 to 25 kg/m^2, an overweight BMI is between 25 and 30 kg/m^2, and obesity is a BMI of greater than 30 kg/m^2. It should be noted, however, that this is not an exact measurement because individuals with a greater muscle mass may have an increased BMI but lack the increased risk of morbidity and mortality.[11] The US Preventive Services Task Force recommends screening all adults for obesity and offering intervention in those who have a BMI in the obese range.[14]

Benefits, Barriers, and Strategies for Treatment

Although obesity continues to be a growing problem, there are a multitude of barriers facing patients regarding weight loss.[15,16] Various life transitions have proven to be barriers to weight loss, including student status, employment, family structure, and health status.[17] Additionally, life stress and significant life events are associated with weight gain.[18] Self-monitoring, social cues, holidays, low physical activity, time management, chronic stress, illness, and internal cues such as thoughts and mood have also been determined to be barriers to weight loss and engaging in physical activity.[19]

Discussing lifestyle modifications in detail and making treatment plans with patients can yield positive results. Studies have shown that the advice physicians give regarding diet and exercise can have a positive influence on patient lifestyle modifications.[20] Studies have also shown that the diagnosis of overweight or obesity and the discussion of this diagnosis can lead to the formulation of treatment plans and a more realistic perception of the patient's own weight and desire to lose weight.[21,22] Despite the benefits of making a diagnosis of obesity with patients, most obese patients have not received a diagnosis and fewer than 50% of primary care physicians report recording BMI consistently.[23,24]

Lifestyle modifications are the mainstay and cornerstone of treatment of obesity and include components such as a reduced calorie meal plan and increased physical activity, along with a combination of behavioral interventions to promote adherence.[25] Treatment for weight loss can be most effective when delivered as a structured program with accommodations for personal and cultural preferences. Primary or specialty care providers, health educators, dietitians, nurses, exercise trainers, and psychologists can all play a role in delivering structured lifestyle interventions.[25]

Examples of healthy meal plans include low carbohydrate, low fat, low glycemic index, DASH, Mediterranean, and vegetarian. The use of meal substitutes in the form of shakes and bars add structure to the diet and have been shown to be effective. The patient should also be instructed in approaches to portion and stimulus control. Commercial programs featuring meal substitutes or delivered meals have also been shown to be effective.[25] Various professional groups have made recommendations regarding diets for weight loss and/or morbidity risk reduction, which can be challenging to physicians when making recommendations to patients. Plans should be individualized to the patient based on risk factors, comorbidities,[26–30] and preferences. **Table 3** provides summaries of these recommendations.

Table 3 Recommendation summaries		
Organization	**Diet**	**Physical Activity**
AHA	Low saturated fat Low *trans* fat High in fruits, vegetables, fish, low-fat dairy, and poultry	Three to four 40-minute sessions per week involving moderate-to-vigorous intensity.
ADA	Individualized. May include DASH diet, low carbohydrate, low fat, Mediterranean, vegan, or vegetarian	150 min of moderate intensity such as brisk walking every week
AACE	45%–65% of ingested energy from carbohydrates 15%–35% from protein 25%–35% from fats	150 min of moderate intensity and strength training
HHS	Variety, nutrient dense; limit calories from added sugars, saturated fats, and *trans* fats	150 min of moderate-intensity or 75 min of vigorous-intensity aerobic activity

Abbreviations: AACE, American Association of Clinical Endocrinologists; ADA, American Diabetes Association; AHA, American Heart Association; HHS, US Department of Health and Human Services.
   Data from Refs.[26–30]

Wearable fitness trackers, smartphone applications, and other devices have allowed for technological integration of weight management with our daily lives. There are some concerns about how well these applications apply evidence-based strategies to help with weight loss.[31] Technology can be an integral part of a patient's personalized lifestyle modification plan, and recommendations should be to use high-quality applications and to use features fully to achieve optimal results.[32]

MENTAL HEALTH
Morbidity and Mortality

The National Institute of Mental Health estimates 1 in 6 US adults lives with mental illness.[33] In the 2016 National Survey on Drug Use and Health, young adults ages 18 to 25 years demonstrated the highest prevalence of having any mental illness (22.1%), followed by adults aged 26 to 49 years (21.1%), and adults aged 50 and older (14.5%); women (48.8%) were more affected than men (33.9%).[34] Various available treatment options include several levels of inpatient or outpatient therapy and/or pharmacotherapy. Yet only 19.2 million of the 44.7 million adults who struggle with mental illness received some form of mental health treatment in 2016.[34] Although higher levels of mental illness are reported among younger adults (ages 18–25), only 35.1% received treatment, which is lower than adults ages 26 to 49 (43.1%) and adults ages 50 and older (46.8%).[34]

Those who are affected by mental illness often suffer unnecessarily owing to limited access to appropriate services and/or a lack of awareness of the availability of treatment options within their community.[35] Primary care physicians are often the first resource for patients seeking help in identifying problematic symptoms and inquiring about treatment options.[36] As a result, primary care physicians are encouraged to have a working knowledge regarding symptoms, screening tools, and treatment options available to their patients.

Benefits, Barriers, and Strategies for Treatment

Screening is an essential part of identifying the presence of mental illness and guiding the treatment approach.[37] Mental health screening tools are brief approaches to collecting information that can be completed at any time during an office visit. Some of the most popular screening tools include the Patient Health Questionnaire, the Generalized Anxiety Disorder questionnaire, and the Mood Disorder Questionnaire.[38–40] It is also recommended to assess for the presence of alcohol and recreational drug misuse using screeners such as the Alcohol Use Disorders Identification Test[41] and the Drug Abuse Screening Test-10.[42] These self-report measures can be critical to engaging patients to participate in early interventions to prevent increased symptom severity.

Although patients with moderate to severe symptoms may require intensive outpatient or inpatient treatment, patients experiencing mild symptoms may benefit from lifestyle modifications and incorporating psychotherapy, counseling, and/or medication therapy aimed at addressing maladaptive thoughts and behaviors and improving approaches to stress relief. Physicians are encouraged to use motivational interviewing to better understand where patients prefer to create change in their lives and partner with patients to implement change. Change can often be guided through self-help resources such as texts and national organization websites, which are readily available to all. Therefore, physicians should speak with mental health professionals to identify appropriate resources for patients. Additionally, patients are encouraged to incorporate a short relaxation routine or mindfulness exercise each day to assist with managing challenging thoughts and mood.[43] Some strategies include not checking e-mail until arriving at work, setting firm boundaries with time spent at work, and using technology like mobile meditation applications to help develop more relaxing habits. Physicians can also help patients to identify barriers in engaging with activities of pleasure and help develop small steps toward engaging in increased activity levels.[43]

When working with patients with more significant symptoms, physicians are encouraged to be aware of treatment providers and programs in their community. An increasing trend in medicine is providing integrative care with a mental health professional within primary care settings. The American Psychological Association encourages psychologists to function in a multidisciplinary position to address health promotion, disease prevention, and primary care, including the care of acute and chronic medical conditions, and has established guidelines for psychological practice in health care systems.[44] Mental health professionals provide services such as brief, consultation-style interventions all the way to traditional individual therapy. Incorporating mental health providers in primary care settings increases the likelihood of patients engaging in psychotherapy, decreasing the perceived stigma felt, and providing improved patient satisfaction scores.[45]

ALCOHOL USE DISORDERS
Morbidity and Mortality

Alcohol misuse has long been tied to a number of health issues, including disorders of the liver, unborn fetus, central nervous system, and cardiovascular system. Despite this widespread knowledge, 15.1 million adults ages 18 and older (6.2% of this age group) are diagnosed with an alcohol use disorder (AUD).[46,47] This includes 9.8 million men and 5.3 million women.[46,48] In 2010, alcohol misuse cost US$249 billion; three-quarters of the total cost of alcohol misuse is related to binge drinking.[48–50] The Substance Abuse and Mental Health Services Administration defines binge drinking as 5 or more alcoholic drinks for males or 4 or more alcoholic drinks for females on the same occasion (ie, at the same time or within a couple of hours of each other) on at least 1 day in the past month.[51]

Benefits, Barriers, and Strategies for Treatment

There are a number of barriers that exist in treating patients on the spectrum of AUD; some are unique to the circumstances around alcohol consumption, and some are borne out of patient misconceptions. Alcohol use is generally considered to be socially acceptable and a large part of the culture in the United States. Additionally, there is an attitudinal barrier to seeking care in alcohol abuse (perceived lack of efficacy; believing problem would "get better on its own" or you "should be able to handle it").[52] There are even more hurdles to overcome with individuals who have comorbid mood disorders and AUD. This comorbidity is common, with some studies showing that 20% of individuals with a mood disorder and 18% of individuals with an anxiety disorder also had a substance use disorder.[53] Interestingly, although these patients perceive a need for treatment, they often feel these needs are not met, most commonly owing to financial barriers.[52] To help patients overcome these barriers, physicians should first identify that such comorbidities exist through use of appropriate screening tools (the Patient Health Questionnaire-2 and -9 for depression, the Generalized Anxiety Disorder-7 questionnaire for anxiety, and the Alcohol Use Disorders Identification Test-C for alcohol use).[54] After screening is complete, physicians can help patients to find programs that address the comorbid conditions (counseling for the mood disorder, support groups such as Alcoholics Anonymous for AUD) or, in severe cases, referral to specialty centers that treat comorbid disorders.[55,56] Something simple physicians can do is suggest activities where social support is present but there is no drinking involved, such as starting a new exercise routine with a friend or practicing a hobby such as mindfulness.

THE OPIOID EPIDEMIC

Every day, more than 115 Americans die after overdosing on opioids.[57] The Centers for Disease Control and Prevention estimates that the total economic burden of prescription opioid misuse alone in the United States is $78.5 billion per year, including the costs of health care, lost productivity, addiction treatment, and criminal justice involvement.[58] A large percentage of patients who abuse opioids do so with prescription drugs: roughly 21% to 29% of patients prescribed opioids for chronic pain misuse them and it is estimated that 80% of patients who use heroin have transitioned to it after prescription opioid use.[49,59]

Defining the issue is also challenging: definitions of abuse and misuse vary, but generally misuse of opioids is a broad term that captures any use outside of prescription parameters, including misunderstanding of instructions, self-medication for sleep or mood symptoms, and compulsive use driven by an opioid use disorder, whereas abuse is an older term that often refers to use of a substance for the feelings elicited during use.[60]

Benefits, Barriers, and Strategies for Treatment

This crisis does not discriminate; it is just as prevalent and deadly in rural America as it is in the urban metropolises that dot our landscape.[61] Owing to this diversity, patient barriers to treatment for opioid use disorders are also widespread: patient fears of uncontrolled pain and the stigma of being labeled as an addict often preclude patients from seeking care. Additional barriers such as comorbid substance abuse disorders or the simple emotional euphoria associated with opioid use also often stop patients in their tracks.[62] In this seemingly overwhelming battle, there are tools physicians have to help their patients. Like all large tasks, taking small steps on an individual level will lead to larger changes. First, if you are a prescriber with a Drug Enforcement Agency waiver for prescribing buprenorphine (which is used for treatment of opioid use disorders), consider using it and educating your patients on the availability of naloxone for opioid overdoses. Studies have shown that more than one-half of those physicians possessing Drug Enforcement Agency waivers are not actually treating patients with opioid use disorders.[63] Second, like many other disorders we treat, destigmatize the disease. Let patients know your office is a judgment-free zone and encourage them to be honest. Despite the US Preventive Services Task Force indeterminate recommendation, routinely screening for substance abuse disorders with scales such as the Drug Abuse Screening Test-10 will help to identify those patients in need of treatment.[64,65] Third, like all major health crises, we must continue to advocate for policy change, both on a grassroots and on a larger level. Be mindful of advocacy opportunities through professional organizations (such as the American Academy of Family Physicians, American College of Osteopathic Family Physicians, and the American Medical Association), as well as opportunities for further education for yourself and patients.

SUMMARY

By addressing tobacco abuse, obesity, mental health, and substance abuse issues through routine screenings and ongoing guidance in the office, physicians will be able to assist patients in making lifestyle changes and accessing necessary therapies for overall improvements in their quality of life. Additionally, by taking the time to understand the common barriers patients impose on themselves when struggling with lifestyle changes and providing patients with resources in your community, you will empower them to take positive steps forward in treatment.

REFERENCES

1. Okuyemi KS, Nollen NL, Ahluwalia JS. Interventions to facilitate smoking cessation. Am Fam Physician 2006;74(2):262–71.
2. US Preventive Services Task Force (USPSTF). Final recommendation statement. Tobacco smoking cessation in adults, including pregnant women: behavioral and pharmacotherapy interventions. Available at: https://www.uspreventive servicestaskforce.org/Page/Document/RecommendationStatementFinal/tobacco-use-in-adults-and-pregnant-women-counseling-and-interventions1. Accessed March 15, 2018.
3. World Health Organization (WHO). WHO report on the global tobacco epidemic 2011. Available at: http://www.who.int/tobacco/global_report/2011/en/. Accessed March 14, 2018.
4. Fast facts and fact sheets. Centers for Disease Control and Prevention (CDC); 2017. Available at: https://www.cdc.gov/tobacco/data_statistics/fact_sheets/index.htm. Accessed March 14, 2018.
5. US Department of Health and Human Services. The health consequences of smoking-50 years of progress: a report of the surgeon general, 2014. Available at: SurgeonGeneral.gov; https://www.surgeongeneral.gov/library/reports/50-years-of-progress/index.html. Accessed March 14, 2018.
6. Jha P, Ramasundarahettige C, Landsman V, et al. 21st-century hazards of smoking and benefits of cessation in the United States. N Engl J Med 2013;368(4):341–50.
7. Larzelere MM, Williams DE. Promoting smoking cessation. Am Fam Physician 2012;85(6):591–8.
8. Finucane MM, Stevens GA, Cowan MJ, et al. National, regional, and global trends in body-mass index since 1980: systematic analysis of health examination surveys and epidemiological studies with 960 country-years and 9.1 million participants. Lancet 2011;377(9765):557–67.
9. Fryar CD, Carroll MD, Ogden CL. Prevalence of Overweight, Obesity, and Extreme Obesity Among Adults Aged 20 and Over: United States, 1960–1962 Through 2013–2014. Atlanta (GA): CDC, National Center for Health Statistics. Available at: https://www.cdc.gov/nchs/data/hestat/obesity_adult_13_14/obesity_adult_13_14.htm. Published July 18, 2016. Accessed January 20, 2018.
10. Kushner RF. Evaluation and management of obesity. In: Kasper D, Fauci A, Hauser S, et al, editors. Harrison's principles of internal medicine. 19th edition. New York: McGraw-Hill; 2014. Available at: http://accessmedicine.mhmedical.com.ezproxy.rowan.edu/content.aspx?bookid=1130&sectionid=79752839. Accessed January 20, 2018.
11. Flier JS, Maratos-Flier E. Biology of obesity. In: Kasper D, Fauci A, Hauser S, et al, editors. Harrison's principles of internal medicine. 19th edition. New York: McGraw-Hill; 2014. Available at: http://accessmedicine.mhmedical.com.ezproxy.rowan.edu/content.aspx?bookid=1130&sectionid=79752768. Accessed January 20, 2018.

12. Calle EE, Rodriguez C, Walker-Thurmond K, et al. Overweight, obesity, and mortality from cancer in a prospectively studied cohort of U.S. adults. N Engl J Med 2003;348:1625–38.

13. Xu JQ, Murphy SL, Kochanek KD, et al. Mortality in the United States, 2015. NCHS data brief, no 267. Hyattsville (MD): National Center for Health Statistics; 2016.

14. Final Recommendation Statement: Weight Loss to Prevent Obesity-Related Morbidity and Mortality in Adults: Behavioral Interventions. Rockville (MD). U.S. Preventive Services Task Force. September 2018. Available at: https://www.uspreventiveservicestaskforce.org/Page/Document/RecommendationStatement Final/obesity-in-adults-interventions1. Accessed November 17, 2018.

15. Stevens J, Truesdale KP, McClain JE, et al. The definition of weight maintenance. Int J Obes (Lond) 2006;30:391–9.

16. Lyznicki JM, Young DC, Riggs JA, et al, Council on Scientific Affairs, American Medical Association. Obesity: assessment and management in primary care. Am Fam Physician 2001;63:2185–96.

17. Metzgar CJ, Preston AG, Miller DL, et al. Facilitators and barriers to weight loss and weight loss maintenance: a qualitative exploration. J Hum Nutr Diet 2015; 28(6):593–603.

18. Elfhag K,, Rossner S. Who succeeds in maintaining weight loss? A conceptual review of factors associated with weight loss maintenance and weight regain. Obes Rev 2005;6:67–85.

19. Venditti EM, Wylie-Rosett J, Delahanty LM, et al, Diabetes Prevention Program Research Group. Short and long-term lifestyle coaching approaches used to address diverse participant barriers to weight loss and physical activity adherence. Int J Behav Nutr Phys Act 2014;11:16.

20. Kreuter MW, Chheda SG, Bull FC. How does physician advice influence patient behavior? Evidence for a priming effect. Arch Fam Med 2000;9:426–33.

21. Post RE, Mainous AG, Gregorie SH, et al. The influence of physician acknowledgement of patients' weight status on patient perceptions of overweight and obesity in the United States. Arch Intern Med 2011;171:316–21.

22. Bardia A, Holtan SG, Slezak JM, et al. Diagnosis of obesity by primary care physicians and impact on obesity management. Mayo Clin Proc 2007;82:927–32.

23. Bleich SN, Bennett WL, Gudzune KA, et al. National survey of US primary care physicians' perspectives about causes of obesity and solutions to improve care. BMJ Open 2012;2:e001871.

24. Smith AW, Borowski LA, Liu B, et al. U.S. primary care physicians' diet, physical activity, and weight-related care of adult patients. Am J Prev Med 2011 July;41: 33–42.

25. Garvey W, Mechanick JI. Obesity and cardiovascular disease. In: Fuster V, Harrington RA, Narula J, et al, editors. Hurst's the heart, 14th ed. New York: McGraw-Hill. Available at: http://accessmedicine.mhmedical.com.ezproxy.rowan.edu/content.aspx?bookid=2046&sectionid=176573367. Accessed January 21, 2018.

26. Eckel RH, Jakicic JM, Ard JD, et al. 2013 AHA/ACC guideline on lifestyle management to reduce cardiovascular risk. J Am Coll Cardiol 2014;63(25 Part B): 2960–84.

27. Evert AB, Boucher JL, Cypress M, et al. Nutrition therapy recommendations for the management of adults with diabetes. Diabetes Care 2014;37(Suppl 1): S120–43.

28. Gonzalez-Campoy J, Jeor SS, Castorino K, et al. Clinical practice guidelines for healthy eating for the prevention and treatment of metabolic and endocrine diseases in adults: cosponsored by the American Association of Clinical Endocrinologists/the American College of Endocrinology and the Obesity Society. Endocr Pract 2013;19(Supplement 3):1–82.

29. Garber AJ, Abrahamson MJ, Barzilay JI, et al. Consensus statement by the American Association of Clinical Endocrinologists and American College of Endocrinology on the comprehensive type 2 diabetes management algorithm – 2018 executive summary. Endocr Pract 2018;24(1):91–120.

30. US Department of Health and Human Services and US Department of Agriculture. 2015–2020 Dietary guidelines for Americans. 8th edition. 2015. Available at: https://health.gov/dietaryguidelines/2015/guidelines/. Accessed January 21, 2018.

31. Pagoto S, Schneider K, Jojic M, et al. Evidence-based strategies in weight-loss mobile apps. Am J Prev Med 2013;45(5):576–82.

32. Neve M, Morgan PJ, Jones PR, et al. Effectiveness of web-based interventions in achieving weight loss and weight loss maintenance in overweight and obese adults: a systematic review with meta-analysis. Obes Rev 2010;11(4):306–21.

33. Mental illness. Bethesda (MD): National Institute of Mental Health; 2017. Available at: https://www.nimh.nih.gov/health/statistics/mental-illness.shtml. Accessed February 10, 2018.

34. Ahrnsbrak R, Bose J, Hedden SL, et al. Key substance use and mental health indicators in the United States: results from the 2016 national survey on drug use and health. 2017. Available at: Samhsa.gov; https://www.samhsa.gov/data/sites/default/files/NSDUH-FFR1-2016/NSDUH-FFR1-2016.htm. Accessed February 10, 2018.

35. Mental Health America. Mental Health in America: access to care data. Available at: http://www.mentalhealthamerica.net/issues/mental-health-america-access-care-data. Accessed March 10, 2018.

36. Wittchen HU, Muhlig S, Beesdo K. Mental disorders in primary care. Dialogues Clin Neurosci 2003;5(2):115–28. Available at: https://www.ncbi.nlm.nih.gov/pmc/articles/PMC3181625/. Accessed March 10, 2018.

37. Derogatis LR. Screening for psychiatric disorders in primary care settings. In: Maruish ME, editor. Handbook of psychological assessment in primary care settings. 2nd edition. New York: Routledge; 2017. p. 167–92. Available at: https://books.google.co.uk/books?id=_TMIDwAAQBAJ&pg=PA167&lpg=PA167&dq=screening+for+psychiatric+disorders+in+primary+care+settings+derogatis&source=bl&ots=YXJYK9R2yO&sig=ocqK5LHAO8eNcaaLH9rAF96hNgg&hl=en&sa=X&redir_esc=y#v=onepage&q=screening%20for%20psychiatric%20disorders%20in%20primary%20care%20settings%20derogatis&f=false. Accessed March 10, 2018.

38. Spitzer RL, Williams JBW, Kroenke K, et al. Patient Health Questionnaire-9. Available at: http://www.phqscreeners.com/sites/g/files/g10016261/f/201412/PHQ-9_English.pdf. Accessed March 10, 2018.

39. Spitzer RL, Williams JBW, Kroenke K, et al. Generalized anxiety disorder questionnaire. Available at: http://www.phqscreeners.com/sites/g/files/g10016261/f/201412/GAD-7_English.pdfGAD-7. Accessed March 10, 2018.

40. Hirschfeld RMA, Williams JBW, Spitzer RL, et al. Development and validation of a screening instrument for bipolar spectrum disorder: the mood disorder questionnaire. Am J Psychiatry 2000;157(11):1873–5.

41. Babor TF, Higgins-Biddle JC, Saunders JB, et al. AUDIT: the alcohol use disorders identification test-guidelines for use in primary care. 2nd edition. Geneva (Switzerland): World Health Organization; 2001.

42. Skinner HA. The drug abuse screening test. Addict Behav 1982;7(4):363–71.

43. Smith M, Robinson L, Shubin J, Segal J. Coping with depression: tips for overcoming depression one step at a time. 2018. Available at: Helpguide.org. https://www.helpguide.org/articles/depression/coping-with-depression.htm. Accessed March 19, 2018.

44. American Psychological Association. Guidelines for psychological practice in health care delivery systems. Am Psychol 2013;68:1–6.

45. Clatney L, MacDonald H, Shah SM. Mental health care in the primary care setting: family physicians' perspectives. Can Fam Physician 2008;54(6):884–9. Available at: https://www.ncbi.nlm.nih.gov/pmc/articles/PMC2426969/. Accessed March 10, 2018.

46. Substance Abuse and Mental Health Services Administration. Results from the 2015 national Survey on drug use and health: detailed tables. Rockville (MD): Center for Behavioral Health Statistics and Quality; 2016. Available at: https://www.samhsa.gov/data/sites/default/files/NSDUH-DetTabs-2015/NSDUH-DetTabs-2015/NSDUH-DetTabs-2015.htm#tab5-6a. Accessed January 17, 2018.

47. Center for Behavioral Health Statistics and Quality. Key substance use and mental health indicators in the United States: results from the 2015 national Survey on drug use and health. Rockville (MD): Center for Behavioral Health Statistics and Quality; 2016. Available at: https://www.samhsa.gov/data/sites/default/files/NSDUH-FFR1-2015/NSDUH-FFR1-2015/NSDUH-FFR1-2015.pdf. Accessed March 26, 2018.

48. Sacks JJ, Gonzales KR, Bouchery EE, et al. 2010 National and state costs of excessive alcohol consumption. Am J Prev Med 2015;49(5):e73–9.

49. Substance Abuse and Mental Health Services Administration (SAMHSA). 2016 Rockville (MD): National Survey on Drug Use and Health (NSDUH). Table 2.46B—alcohol use, binge alcohol use, and heavy alcohol use in past month among persons aged 12 or older, by demographic characteristics: percentages, 2014 and 2015.

50. Substance Abuse and Mental Health Services Administration. Binge drinking: terminology and patterns of use. Rockville (MD): Substance Abuse and Mental Health Services Administration; 2016. Available at: https://www.samhsa.gov/capt/tools-learning-resources/binge-drinking-terminology-patterns. Accessed March 25, 2018.

51. Kaufmann CN, Chen L-Y, Crum RM, et al. Treatment seeking and barriers to treatment for alcohol use in persons with alcohol use disorders and comorbid mood or anxiety disorders. Soc Psychiatry Psychiatr Epidemiol 2014;49(9):1489–99.

52. Grant BF, Stinson FS, Dawson DA, et al. Prevalence and co-occurrence of substance use disorders and independent mood and anxiety disorders. Arch Gen Psychiatry 2004;61(8):807–16.

53. National Institute on Alcohol Abuse and Alcoholism. Rethinking drinking: alcohol and your health. Bethesda (MD): National Institute on Alcohol Abuse and Alcoholism; 2010.

54. Donovan DM, Ingalsbe MH, Benbow J, et al. 12-step interventions and mutual support programs for substance use disorders: an overview. Soc Work Public Health 2013;28(3–4):313–32.

55. Hedegaard H, Warner M, Miniño AM. Drug overdose deaths in the United States, 1999–2016. NCHS Data Brief, no 294. Hyattsville (MD): National Center for Health Statistics; 2017.

56. Centers for Disease Control and Prevention (CDC). Wide-ranging online data for epidemiologic research (WONDER). Atlanta (GA): CDC, National Center for Health Statistics; 2016.

57. Florence CS, Zhou C, Luo F, et al. The economic burden of prescription opioid overdose, abuse, and dependence in the United States, 2013. Med Care 2016; 54(10):901–6.

58. Vowles KE, Mcentee ML, Julnes PS, et al. Rates of opioid misuse, abuse, and addiction in chronic pain. Pain 2015;156(4):569–76.

59. Muhuri PK, Gfroerer JC, Davies MC. Associations of nonmedical pain reliever use and initiation of heroin use in the United States. CBHSQ data review. 2013. Available at: https://www.samhsa.gov/data/sites/default/files/DR006/DR006/nonmedical-pain-reliever-use-2013.htm. Accessed March 25, 2018.

60. Brady KT, McCauley JL, Back SE. Prescription opioid misuse, abuse, and treatment in the united states: an update. Am J Psychiatry 2016;173(1):18–26.

61. Vivolo-Kantor AM, Seth P, Gladden RM, et al. Vital signs: trends in emergency department visits for suspected opioid overdoses — United States, July 2016–September 2017. MMWR Morb Mortal Wkly Rep 2018;67:279–85.

62. Stumbo SP, Yarborough BJH, McCarty D, et al. Patient-reported pathways to opioid use disorders and pain-related barriers to treatment engagement. J Subst Abuse Treat 2017;73:47–54.

63. Crawford C. Overcoming barriers to opioid treatment takes center stage. AAFP Home; 2017. Available at: https://www.aafp.org/news/health-of-the-public/20170811opioidsstudy.html. Accessed March 21, 2018.

64. Final recommendation statement. Drug use, illicit: screening. US Preventive Services Task Force; 2014. Available at: https://www.uspreventiveservicestaskforce.org/Page/Document/RecommendationStatementFinal/drug-use-illicit-screening. Accessed March 21, 2018.

65. U.S. Preventative Services Task Force. Substance Abuse and Mental Health Services Administration. Rockville (MD): Screening tools. Available at: https://www.integration.samhsa.gov/clinical-practice/screening-tools. Accessed March 21, 2018.

Prescription of Aspirin and Statins in Primary Prevention

Charles H. Hennekens, MD, DrPH[a],*,
Nicole Schuttenberg, BS, MS[a,1], Marc A. Pfeffer, MD, PhD[b]

KEYWORDS

- Cardiovascular disease • Adjunctive drug therapies • Aspirin • Statins
- Metabolic syndrome

KEY POINTS

- Primary care providers must consider multifactorial interventions to address mortality from cardiovascular disease, including therapeutic lifestyle interventions, and adjunctive drug therapies.
- Managing cardiovascular disease risk among primary prevention patients differs from managing secondary prevention risk and requires judgments for individual patients.
- Data from randomized controlled clinical trials can assist primary care providers in informing decisions for individual patients.
- Drug therapies of proven benefit, such as aspirin and statins, should be used as adjuncts, not alternatives, to therapeutic lifestyle changes.

INTRODUCTION

Cardiovascular disease (CVD) is and will remain the leading cause of death in the United States and is rapidly becoming so in most developed countries as well as worldwide.[1] The major components of CVD are myocardial infarction (MI) and stroke, most commonly ischemic. Over many decades in the United States, there have been improvements in life expectancy due chiefly to decreases in mortality from CVD, which, not surprisingly to some, are no longer evident. Specifically, during the last 2 years life expectancy in the United States has been declining and may continue to do so due, in part, to unprecedented epidemics of obesity, physical inactivity, and type 2 diabetes in middle-aged populations as well as young adults. Metabolic

Disclosure Statement: See last page of article.
[a] Charles E. Schmidt College of Medicine, Florida Atlantic University, Boca Raton, FL, USA;
[b] Division of Cardiovascular Medicine, The Harvard Medical School, Brigham and Women's Hospital, 45 Francis Street, Boston, MA 02115, USA
[1] Present address: 2025 Lavers Circle, Delray Beach, FL 33444.
* Corresponding author. 2800 South Ocean Boulevard Apartment PH, Boca Raton, FL 33432.
E-mail address: profchhmd@prodigy.net

Prim Care Clin Office Pract 46 (2019) 13–25
https://doi.org/10.1016/j.pop.2018.10.004
0095-4543/19/© 2018 Elsevier Inc. All rights reserved.
primarycare.theclinics.com

syndrome, a constellation of overweight and obesity that includes dyslipidemia, hypertension, and insulin resistance, a precursor to type 2 diabetes, is becoming increasingly common and is associated with high risks of a first CVD event.[1,2]

Primary health care providers are the backbone of the US health care system and evaluate most primary prevention subjects, specifically, those who have not yet developed CVD, as well as secondary prevention patients, or those who have already experienced manifestations of CVD, especially MI or stroke.[3] Primary prevention subjects with metabolic syndrome constitute about 40% of the US population aged 40 and over and have almost as high a risk of a first CVD event as secondary prevention patients who have already survived a prior event. In the United States as well as other developed and developing countries, metabolic syndrome is becoming the new "silent killer," a term used decades earlier to characterize hypertension. Primary health care providers should be aware of the need for multifactorial interventions, which include therapeutic lifestyle changes (TLCs) as well as adjunctive drug therapies of proven benefit. TLCs of proven benefit include principally avoidance and cessation of cigarette smoking, overweight and obesity, and engaging in regular physical activity.

For a disease as common and serious as CVD, drugs of proven value are likely to have absolute benefits that outweigh their absolute risks in primary prevention subjects at sufficient risk of a first CVD event. In other words, the clinical challenge for primary health care providers is to decide for each subject, whether his or her absolute benefit-to-risk ratio for the primary prevention of CVD will tend to be favorable. Furthermore, the reliable detection of the most plausible small to moderate benefits of adjunctive drug therapies in primary prevention requires data from large-scale randomized trials designed a priori to test the hypothesis and their meta-analyses.[4,5] In this article, the authors review the randomized evidence concerning aspirin and statins as adjunctive drug therapies to TLCs in primary prevention. Our goal is to provide guidance for primary health care providers in their clinical decision making to maximize benefit and minimize harm.

Aspirin

In secondary prevention, the absolute benefits of aspirin are large in relation to the absolute risks, which are, primarily, major extracranial bleeding. Hemorrhagic stroke is very serious but very rare. The absolute benefit on first coronary events, principally MI and stroke, is about 20%, and the absolute risks of major extracranial bleeding, principally gastrointestinal (GI), range from about 1% in young and middle age to about 4% in older individuals.[6]

In primary prevention, the US Physicians' Health Study (PHS) was the first randomized trial to demonstrate that aspirin significantly reduces the risk of a first MI.[7,8] A total of 22,071 dedicated and conscientious, apparently healthy male physicians aged 40 to 84 years were randomized to either 325-mg aspirin on alternate days or placebo. The trial was stopped early based on the unanimous recommendation of the independent Data and Safety Monitoring Board (DSMB) due principally to the emergence of a statistically extreme ($P<.0001$) 44% reduction in risk of a first MI. With respect to gender, the totality of the randomized evidence indicates no differences in response to aspirin between men and women.[9]

A comprehensive meta-analysis of 6 major published randomized trials of aspirin in primary prevention was performed by the Antithrombotic Trialists' Collaboration (ATT).[6] These analyses included individual patient level data among more than 95,000 men and women randomly assigned to aspirin at doses between 75 and 500 mg per day, placebo, or open control. In the ATT meta-analysis, aspirin significantly reduced major coronary events, strokes, and all serious vascular events[6]

(**Table 1**). These relative risk reductions in various CVD events in primary prevention were similar to those in secondary prevention. Nonetheless, in all these major primary prevention trials, the average absolute risk was less than 5%. In the ATT meta-analyses, about 80,000 of the approximately 95,000 randomized subjects, or nearly 80%, were low-risk subjects in the PHS of 22,071 men, the Women's Health Study of 39,876 women, and the Hypertension Optimal Treatment Trial of 18,790 men and women. In each of these 3 trials, the 10-year risks of a first coronary event were 4.8%, 2.5%, and 3.6%, respectively (**Table 2**).[6] All these estimates are far lower than the 10-year risk of a first event of 10%, which is the level generally used to define moderate risk primary as well as the threshold for deciding about whether to prescribe aspirin for primary prevention subjects.[10–12]

In addition, the primary health care provider should be aware that a 20% relative risk reduction in a patient with a 10-year risk of a first coronary event of 5% is about 1%. Similarly, a 10% relative risk reduction in a patient with a 10-year risk of a first coronary event of 5% is about 0.5%. Furthermore, if one assumes that the risk of a bleeding event is the same as in secondary prevention, then, based on the small amount of randomized evidence available in moderate-risk subjects, the benefits will tend to outweigh the risks only when the risk of a first coronary event begins to exceed 10% in 10 years. In addition, in the ATT meta-analysis, age is a risk factor for bleeding as well as occlusion. Finally, not all patients are at equal risk for the development of major bleeding. For example, patients with a history of GI bleed, those on chronic nonsteroidal anti-inflammatory drugs, and those with GI symptoms attributable to or history of ulcer disease, gastritis, or gastroesophageal reflux disease are all at increased risks of major bleeding.[10–12]

At present, there are insufficient numbers of moderate-risk primary prevention subjects in the trials to provide a rational basis upon which to make any general guidelines for the use of aspirin in primary prevention. In addition, primary health care providers should remain cognizant that individual clinical decision making for aspirin in the primary prevention of CVD is far more complex than that for secondary prevention.[10–12] Based on all these aforementioned considerations, in primary prevention, aspirin should be prescribed only when based on an individual clinical judgment and only when the magnitude of the absolute benefit exceeds the magnitude of the absolute risk.

Table 1 Aspirin in the secondary and primary prevention of cardiovascular diseases	
	Risk Ratios (95% Confidence Intervals)
Major coronary events	
Secondary prevention	0.80 (0.72, 0.92)
Primary prevention	0.82 (0.75, 0.90)
Strokes	
Secondary prevention	0.78 (0.61, 0.99)
Primary prevention	0.86 (0.74, 1.00)
All serious vascular events	
Secondary prevention	0.81 (0.75, 0.87)
Primary prevention	0.88 (0.82, 0.94)

Data from Antithrombotic Trialists (ATT) Collaboration. Aspirin in the primary and secondary prevention of vascular disease: collaborative meta-analysis of individual participant data from randomised trials. Lancet. 2009;373:1853.

Table 2	
Low 10-y risk of a first coronary event among randomized participants in the 6 major primary prevention trials of aspirin in the Antithrombotic Trialists' Collaboration meta-analysis	
WHS	2.5%
HOT	3.6%
PPP	4.3%
PHS	4.8%
BMD	8.9%
TPT	12.4%

Data from Antithrombotic Trialists (ATT) Collaboration. Aspirin in the primary and secondary prevention of vascular disease: collaborative meta-analysis of individual participant data from randomised trials. Lancet 2009;373:1849–60.

When the magnitude of benefit is similar to that of risk, patient preference, which is always a consideration, will increase. For example, a primary prevention subject who feels that the prevention of a first MI or stroke is more important than the development of a GI bleed may state a clear preference for aspirin use. Such an approach, however, may not be as useful in subjects at higher risks of bleeding. Primary health care providers should be aware that many primary prevention subjects are at a moderate to high risk of a first CVD event. These include the approximately 40% of the US population aged 40 and over with metabolic syndrome, whose 10-year risks of a first CVD event are as high as 16% to 18%.[2]

Very recently, the results of three large scale trials of aspirin in primary prevention in subjects at moderate risk have been reported. The A Study of Cardiovascular Events iN Diabetes (ASCEND) trial randomized 15,480 subjects at least 40 years of age with diabetes and showed a statistically significant benefit on major vascular events (RR=0.88, 95%CI 0.79-0.97,p=0.010).[13] The Aspirin to Reduce Risk of Initial Vascular Events (ARRIVE) trial randomized 12,546 subjects over age 55 for men and over age 60 for women with moderate cardiovascular risk and showed no significant reduction in first occurrence of a primary pre-specified combined CVD event (HR=0.96;95%CI 0.81-1.13).[14] Finally, the Aspirin in Reducing Events in the Elderly (ASPREE) trial randomized 18,117 subjects over age 70 and showed no significant reduction in the primary pre-specified combined CVD endpoint (HR=0.95;95%CI 0.83-1.08).[15] It may be of importance to note that follow up rates were far higher in ASCEND than in either ARRIVE or ASPREE.[13–15] Perhaps of even greater importance, adherence rates were about 70% in both groups in ASCEND and about 60% in both groups in ASPREE. These data refer to average adherence over the course of the trial whereas the most informative data would derive from the later years of follow up where the majority of the endpoints accrue. These methodologic differences may, at least, in part, explain the apparently the failure to detect a small to moderate benefit in older subjects at moderate risk in ARRIVE or ASPREE in contrast to the previously reported significant benefits in older subjects at lower risks in the PHS, WHS and the ATT meta analysis. Nonadherence is a particularly large potential source of bias in trials of aspirin as the half life of the platelet is about 8 days which is why those on aspirin undergoing elective surgery are asked to stop the drug for at least one week. Finally, it might be helpful to understand the interrelationships of aspirin and statin use with adherence and follow up. All these considerations emphasize the crucial importance to conduct another worldwide meta-analysis of trials using individual participant data which would shed light on whether, and, if so, which of these methodologic limitations influenced the overall results. Another trial in moderate risk primary prevention subjects,

> **Box 1**
> **Rationale for additive benefits of statins and aspirin to decrease risks of cardiovascular disease**
>
> *Atherosclerosis*
> The principal underlying cause of occlusive CVD events, which is inhibited by statins
>
> *Thrombosis*
> The principal proximate cause of occlusive CVD events, which is inhibited by aspirin
>
> *Data from* Hebert PR, Pfeffer MA, Hennekens CH. Use of statins and aspirin to reduce cardio-vascular disease. J Cardiovasc Pharmacol Ther 2002;7:77–80.

the Aspirin and Simvastatin Combination for Cardiovascular Events Prevention Trials in Diabetes (ACCEPT-D) trials, is still ongoing.[16] Primary health care providers should note that the National Cholesterol Education Program Adult Treatment Panel III elevated diabetes from a risk factor to a CHD risk equivalent.[17] Using this approach, all primary prevention patients with diabetes should be treated like secondary prevention patients who have survived a prior CVD event. This rationale derived, in part, from earlier consistent observational study data that patients with long-standing diabetes have several-fold increased risks of CHD, which are even greater in women than men. This rationale, however, did not consider that a sufficient duration may have to accrue before subjects with new onset diabetes accrue higher risks of CVD.

With respect to aspirin and statins, it was tempting to speculate that the benefits on CVD endpoints would be additive. Aspirin primarily affects thrombosis, the principal proximate cause, and statins primarily affect atherosclerosis, the principal underlying cause of clinical CVD events (**Box 1**).[18] Randomized data on statins and observational data on aspirin demonstrate, at the very least, additive benefits on all clinical CVD end-points (**Fig. 1**).[19] In fact, in these data, the probability of synergy between aspirin and statins is 0.92.[20]

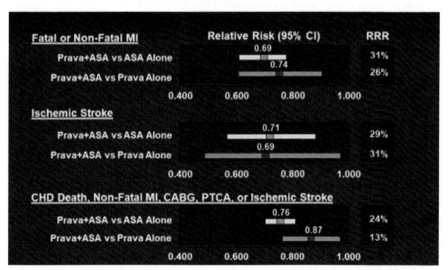

Fig. 1. Greater relative risk reductions for pravastatin + ASA versus pravastatin or ASA alone. ASA, aspirin; CABG, coronary artery bypass grafting; CHD, coronary heart disease; PTCA, percutaneous transluminal coronary angioplasty. (*Data from* Hennekens CH, Sacks F, Tonkin A, et al. Additive benefits of pravastatin and aspirin to decrease risks of cardiovascular disease: randomized and observational comparisons of secondary prevention trials and their meta-analysis. Arch Intern Med 2004;164:40–4; with permission.)

Recently, increased attention has focused on the possible role of aspirin in the primary prevention of cancer. There is a large body of basic research and observational epidemiologic studies suggesting that individuals who self-select for aspirin use have reductions in several different cancers. These observational data, however, are useful only to generate hypotheses but are unreliable to test hypotheses of the most plausible small to moderate benefits.[4,5] In randomized data, one trial showed significant benefits of aspirin in reducing adenomas in patients with prior colorectal cancer (CRC), and another demonstrated significant benefits in reducing recurrent adenomas in primary prevention subjects.[21,22] As regards aspirin in the primary prevention of CRC, there are no large-scale individual trials designed a priori to test the hypothesis. There are, however, meta-analyses of trials of aspirin in primary prevention of CVD suggesting that aspirin reduces risks of CRC. The US Preventive Services Task Force (USPSTF) used a microsimulation model taking into consideration baseline risk factors and aspirin utilization to provide an estimate of CVD event rates. This included nonfatal MIs, ischemic stroke, and cases of CRC prevented by aspirin, which was stratified by risk score, sex, and age, along with major extracranial bleeds. The USPSTF considered 11 randomized trials of CVD in conjunction with 3 primary and secondary prevention trials of CVD to conclude that long-term use of aspirin is associated with a 40% reduction in CRC. The specific recommendations of the USPSTF are as follows[23]:

1. Patients aged less than 50: Unable to evaluate benefits versus risks. No recommendation made.
2. Patients aged 50 to 59: Highest benefit group for daily low-dose aspirin (81 mg) if CVD risk is greater than 10%, because benefits outweigh the harms if they do not have any other factors that would predispose them to bleeding. In addition, this group is more likely to experience benefit for CRC prevention due to life expectancy if they are willing to comply with daily aspirin therapy.
3. Patients aged 60 to 69: Likely to benefit from aspirin therapy if CVD risk score is 10% or higher, because they are still expected to have a favorable benefit versus risk outlook. However, this group is less likely to experience benefit in regards to CRC prevention.
4. Patients aged 70 or greater: Unable to evaluate benefits versus risks. No recommendation made.
5. No gender-specific recommendations were supported with respect to the above.

The absolute risk of colon cancer alone, however, is not sufficiently high to warrant the absolute risk of side effects from aspirin. Based on the totality of evidence, primary health care providers may wish to consider aspirin prophylaxis when the absolute risk of colon cancer is higher, such as in primary prevention subjects with a positive family history. Because the risk factors for colon cancer are similar to those for CVD, those at higher risk also include primary prevention subjects with other major risk factors, such as overweight or obesity and physical inactivity.[12]

Statins

Numerous large-scale trials in secondary and primary prevention demonstrate that individuals assigned randomly to statins have statistically significant and clinically important reductions in risks of various manifestations of CVD. Several comprehensive worldwide meta-analyses using individual patient data have been performed by the Cholesterol Lowering Trialists' Collaboration (CTT) of statins in high-, moderate-, and low-risk subjects, including those without prior CVD events. These analyses have demonstrated clinical benefits of statins on MI, stroke, as well as CVD and total

Table 3
Proportional effects on total and cause-specific mortality per millimole per liter (38 mg/dL) reduction in low-density lipoprotein cholesterol: 26 randomized trials of statins with 169,138 participants

Cause of Death	Statin (n = 84,573) (Events [%] per Annum)	Control (n = 84,565) (Events [%] per Annum)	Relative Risk (95% Confidence Interval)
All cause	2.1	2.3	0.90 (0.87–0.93)
Coronary heart disease	0.5	0.6	0.80 (0.74–0.87)
Other cardiac	0.4	0.5	0.89 (0.81–0.98)
Stroke	0.1	0.1	0.96 (0.84–1.09)
Other vascular	0.1	0.1	0.98 (0.81–1.18)
Any vascular	1.2	1.3	0.86 (0.82–0.90)
Any nonvascular	0.8	0.8	0.97 (0.92–1.03)
Cancer	0.5	0.5	0.99 (0.91–1.09)

Data from Cholesterol Treatment Trialists' (CTT) Collaboration. Efficacy and safety of more intensive lowering of LDL cholesterol: a meta-analysis of data from 170,000 participants in 26 randomized trials. Lancet. 2010;376:1677.

mortality[24–29] (**Table 3**). The most recent CTT meta-analysis focused on low-risk primary prevention subjects and included data from 2 different trial designs.[29] Of 27 trials, 22 compared statin versus control involving 134,537 subjects with a median follow-up of 4.8 years. In these trials, subjects randomized to statins achieved a mean difference in low-density lipoprotein cholesterol (LDL-C) of about 40 mg/dL, which translates to approximately 1.03 mmol/L. In addition, 5 trials compared more versus less statin involving 39,612 subjects with a mean follow-up of 5.1 years and a mean LDL-C difference of about 20 mg/dL (0.52 mmol/L). In low-risk primary prevention subjects, defined as those with a 10-year risk of major coronary events less than 10%, each 39 mg/dL (1.0 mmol/L) reduction in LDL-C produced an absolute reduction in major vascular events of about 11 per 1000 over 5 years. This absolute benefit greatly exceeds any known risks of statin therapy. Finally, the lower the LDL-C, the greater the clinical benefit, and there was no apparent threshold below which there was no incremental benefit (**Table 4**).[24,30]

In the primary prevention of CVD with statins, the largest, and perhaps most informative, individual trial is the Justification for the Use of Statins in Prevention: an Intervention Trial Evaluating Rosuvastatin (JUPITER), in which 17,802 primary prevention subjects without elevated LDL-C levels were randomized to either a daily dose of 20 mg rosuvastatin or placebo.[31] These primary prevention subjects had a 10-year risk of a first event of about 16% and, not surprisingly, 41% had metabolic syndrome. Inflammation plays a seminal role in the pathogenesis of atherosclerosis and is assessed by high-sensitivity C-reactive protein (hs-CRP) greater than 2.0 mg/L, a sensitive marker for CVD.[32] In JUPITER, the selection criterion of risk was an elevation of hs-CRP rather than an increase in LDL. At baseline, randomized subjects had LDL-C levels of about 108 mg/dL (2.82 mmol/L), which are levels that would not have generally led clinicians to prescribe statins based on the existing US guidelines.[17] Following randomization, the achieved LDL-C levels were 55 mg/dL (1.42 mmol/L) in the rosuvastatin group and remained at 108 mg/dL (2.82 mmol/L) in the placebo group. The trial was terminated early after 1.9 years of a 5-year scheduled duration, based on the unanimous recommendation of the independent DSMB. Randomized subjects assigned to 20 mg rosuvastatin daily compared with placebo

Table 4		
Clinical guidance for prescription of evidence-based doses of statins in primary prevention		
Risk of Patient	Atorvastatin, mg	Rosuvastatin, mg
High	80	40
Moderate	20–40	10–20
Low	10–20	5–10

There is no level of LDL below which there are no incremental benefits
- Randomized data showing clinical CVD benefits primarily in patients treated with statins
- Randomized data showing incremental benefits of statins achieve LDL levels of 50–60 mg/dL
- Population data from Japan suggest that individuals with LDLs of 50 mg/dL have higher life expectancies

Data from Hennekens CH, Lieberman E, Rubenstein M, et al. Lipid modification in the treatment and prevention of cardiovascular diseases: emerging clinical and public health challenges. In: Watson RR, editor. Handbook of cholesterol. Urbana (IL): AOCS Press; 2016. p. 155–81; and Gitin A, Pfeffer MA, Hennekens CH. Editorial commentary: the lower the LDL the better but how and how much? Trends Cardiovasc Med 2018;28(5):355–6.

experienced a statistically extreme (P<.0001) 44% reduction in the primary prespecified combined endpoint of MI, stroke, unstable angina, revascularization, or CVD death as well as the individual components of MI, stroke, and revascularization. In addition, subjects randomized to rosuvastatin experienced a significant 20% decrease in total mortality (P = .02).[32]

The randomized evidence for benefits of statins in primary prevention should be considered in the context of possible adverse effects. Adverse effects from some statins on muscle, such as myopathy with increasing levels of creatine kinase, and rhabdomyolysis, or on the liver, with increasing levels of transaminases, are rare at standard doses. Furthermore, asymptomatic increases in liver transaminases are not clearly associated with an increased risk of liver disease. In fact, metabolic syndrome patients with increases in liver transaminases due to fatty livers tend to achieve normal levels. In randomized, double-blind, placebo-controlled trials and their meta-analyses, statins are safe and well tolerated.[24,30] At present, however, there are large discrepancies between randomized evidence and self-reports by patients of muscle symptoms.[33] Claims data, no matter how large, are useful only to formulate, not test hypotheses. Claims data suggest a positive relationship of statin use with muscle pain but suffer from uncontrolled and uncontrollable confounding.[4,5] In clinical practice, several strategies have been proposed for subjects with statin intolerance. They include discontinuation of the particular statin being prescribed and checking muscle enzymes as well as investigating other causes of elevations. Subsequently, clinicians may wish to consider a different class of statins as lipophilic drugs include atorvastatin, lovastatin, and simvastatin, and hydrophilic drugs include rosuvastatin and pravastatin. Finally, it is possible to consider decreasing the daily dose as well as alternate day, or less frequent dosing. Finally, it is possible to add coenzyme Q10 if that results in less perceived side effects.[30]

The American College of Cardiology/American Heart Association published their most recent Guideline on the Treatment of Blood Cholesterol Adult Treatment Panel IV recommendations. These guidelines identify the following:

1. Secondary prevention patients with prior CVD,
2. Primary prevention subjects with LDL ≥190
3. Primary prevention subjects with diabetes mellitus (DM) aged 40 to 75, with LDL 70 to 189,

4. Primary prevention subjects without DM, aged 40 to 75, with LDL 70 to 189, and a 10-year CVD risk ≥7.5% by risk calculator.[34]

These latter subjects should include low-risk men and women with no previous history of CVD[35] as well as higher-risk patients with DM[36] or chronic kidney disease. The development of diabetes in primary prevention subjects with and without metabolic syndrome will increase their risks of CVD about 2- to 3-fold in men and 4- to 6-fold in women. Triglycerides are considered by some to be an accurate predictor of future diabetes, especially in subjects with metabolic syndrome.[36]

The algorithm used to calculate risk is based on a pooled cohort that included participants from several large racially and geographically diverse US National Heart Lung and Blood Institute–sponsored cohort studies including the Atherosclerosis Risk in Communities Study, the Cardiovascular Health Study, Coronary Artery Risk Development in Young Adults Study combined with applicable data from the Framingham original and offspring study cohorts. Although risk calculator helps clinicians discern between high, moderate, and low risk, precise quantification should be based on the astute judgment of the clinician following a review of the totality of evidence.[37] For example, overweight and obesity as well as physical inactivity are major risk factors for CVD but are not included in the risk algorithm. The new US guidelines have recommended intensive statin therapy up to age 75 and moderate therapy thereafter. Nonetheless, the data from large-scale randomized trials are relatively robust and suggest net benefits up to age 85 regardless of whether there is a prior event. Beyond that age, the absence of data does not necessarily imply the absence of benefit. Some have suggested the need for randomized trials in the oldest old. At present, there is no substitute for astute individual clinical judgment coupled with a consultation with each of his or her patients in the context of the totality of evidence as well as frank discussions of preferences as well as quality of life and costs.[38,39]

In summary, in primary prevention subjects, including those at low to moderate risk, statins produce statistically significant and clinically important reductions in MI, stroke, and CVD as well as total mortality. Any debate about the absolute level at low risk in which to initiate statin therapy should be viewed in the context of the high prevalence of metabolic syndrome, which confers high risks of CVD. More intensive lipid lowering with evidence-based doses of high potency statins produces incremental clinical benefits when compared with usual statin regimens. In all risk categories (high, moderate, or low risk), the size of the proportional reduction in major vascular events is directly proportional to the absolute reduction in LDL-C that is achieved. Finally, there is no threshold for LDL-C below which there are no benefits indicating that patients at high and moderate risk of occlusive vascular events should achieve the largest LDL-C reduction possible.[24] In this regard, in the randomized trials showing incremental benefits achieved, the LDL-C is about 50 to 60, which are approximately the same levels that had been achieved by adult Asian populations before the introduction of the Western diet and lifestyle.[30,39,40] These levels of LDL-C are achievable with evidence-based doses of rosuvastatin or atorvastatin, which should be prescribed with consideration of the absolute risk of the primary prevention subject (see **Table 4**).

SUMMARY

Randomized trials are a necessary component of any guideline. Furthermore, any guideline should provide guidance to the health care provider.[39] In primary prevention, the totality of evidence indicates the clear need for primary health care providers to aggressively use a multifactorial approach in reducing risks of a first CVD event.

Primary health care providers should engage in patient-centered primary prevention to increase their willingness to adopt all TLCs of proven benefit. Drug therapies of proven benefit should be used as adjuncts, not alternatives, to TLCs. Although aspirin and statins are drug therapies of proven benefit and appear to be effective even in the absence of TLCs, their benefits are, at least, additive. At present, the totality of evidence indicates that clinicians should initiate statin therapy and then consider aspirin, on an individual patient basis, if the residual risk of an occlusive event is sufficiently high to warrant the side effects.[12,13,31,39] The implementation of multifactorial interventions, including TLCs as well as aspirin and statins, as adjunctive drug therapies by clinicians for their individual patients and policymakers for the health of the general public can markedly reduce premature morbidity and mortality from CVD, especially in high-risk primary prevention subjects with metabolic syndrome.[38]

The increasing burden of CVD worldwide in developed and developing countries underscores the need for the more widespread use of aspirin and statins as adjunctive drug therapies of proven net benefit in primary prevention of CVD, optimally not as alternatives to TLCs.

DISCLOSURE STATEMENT

Ms N. Schuttenberg has nothing to disclose. Professor M.A. Pfeffer reports that he receives research support from Novartis; serves as a consultant to AstraZeneca, Bayer, Boehringer Ingelheim, DalCor (for which he also holds stock options), Genzyme, Gilead, GlaxoSmithKline, Janssen, Lilly, Novartis, Novo Nordisk, Sanofi, Teva, and Thrasos. Professor C.H. Hennekens reports that he is funded by the Charles E. Schmidt College of Medicine of Florida Atlantic University; serves as an independent scientist in an advisory role to investigators and sponsors as Chair or Member of Data and Safety Monitoring Boards for Amgen, AstraZeneca, British Heart Foundation, Cadila, Canadian Institutes of Health Research, DalCor, and Regeneron; to the Collaborative Institutional Training Initiative; United States Food and Drug Administration, and UpToDate; receives royalties for authorship or editorship of 3 textbooks and as coinventor on patents for inflammatory markers and cardiovascular disease that are held by Brigham and Women's Hospital; has an investment management relationship with the West-Bacon Group within Sun-Trust Investment Services, which has discretionary investment authority; does not own any common or preferred stock in any pharmaceutical or medical device company.

ACKNOWLEDGMENTS

The authors are indebted to Professor Colin Baigent of The Clinical Trial Service and Epidemiology Studies Unit and Nuffield Department of Population Health, Oxford University.

REFERENCES

1. Caldwell M, Martinez L, Foster J, et al. Prospects for the primary prevention of myocardial infarction and stroke. J Cardiovasc Pharmacol Ther 2019; [Epub ahead of print].
2. Sherling DH, Perumareddi P, Hennekens CH. Clinical and policy implications of metabolic syndrome: the new silent killer. J Cardiovasc Pharmacol Ther 2017; 22:365–7.

3. Kohli P, Whelton SP, Hsu S, et al. Clinician's guide to the updated ABCs of cardiovascular disease prevention. J Am Heart Assoc 2014;3(5):e001098.
4. Hennekens CH, DeMets D. The need for large scale randomized evidence without undue emphasis on small trials, meta-analyses or subgroup analyses. JAMA 2009;302:2361–2.
5. Hennekens CH, DeMets D. Statistical association and causation: contributions of different types of evidence. JAMA 2011;306:1134–6.
6. Antithrombotic Trialists' (ATT) Collaboration, Baigent C, Blackwell L, Collins R, et al. Aspirin in the primary and secondary prevention of vascular disease: collaborative meta-analysis of individual participant data from randomised trials. Lancet 2009;373:1849–60.
7. The Steering Committee of the Physicians' Health Study Research Group, Belanger C, Buring JE, Eberlein K, et al. Preliminary report: findings from the aspirin component of the ongoing Physicians' Health Study. N Engl J Med 1988;318:262–4.
8. The Steering Committee of the Physicians' Health Study Research Group, Belanger C, Buring JE, Cook N, et al. Final report on the aspirin component of the ongoing Physicians' Health Study. N Engl J Med 1989;321:129–35.
9. Hennekens CH, Hollar D, Baigent C. Gender differences in response to aspirin in cardiovascular disease: a hypothesis formulated, but not tested. Nat Clin Pract Cardiovasc Med 2006;3:4–5.
10. Hennekens CH, DeMets D. Aspirin in primary prevention needs individual clinical judgements. Nat Rev Cardiol 2014;11:438–40.
11. Hennekens CH, Baigent C. Aspirin in primary prevention: good news and bad news. Nat Rev Cardiol 2012;9:262–3.
12. Hennekens CH, Bjorkman DJ. The risks and benefits of prophylactic aspirin in vascular disease and cancer: what's a doctor to do? Clin Investig 2013;3(5):449.
13. Bayer HealthCare. ARRIVE. Aspirin to reduce risk of initial vascular events. 2012. Available at: http://www.arrive-study.com/EN/study.cfm.
14. Nelson MR, Reid C, Beilin L, et al. Rationale for a trial of low-dose aspirin for the primary prevention of major adverse cardiovascular events and vascular dementia in the elderly. Aspirin in Reducing Events in the Elderly (ASPREE). Drugs Aging 2003;20:897–903.
15. University of Oxford. ASCEND. A study of cardiovascular events in diabetes [online]. 2012. Available at: http://www.ctsu.ox.ac.uk/ascend/.
16. De Berardis G, Sacco M, Evangelista V, et al. Aspirin and Simvastatin Combination for Cardiovascular Events Prevention Trials in Diabetes (ACCEPT-D): design of a randomized study of the efficacy of low-dose aspirin in the prevention of cardiovascular events in subjects with diabetes mellitus treated with statins. Trials 2007;8:21.
17. Expert Panel on Detection, Evaluation, and Treatment of High Blood Cholesterol in Adults. Executive summary of the third report of the National Cholesterol Education Program (NCEP) expert panel on detection, evaluation, and treatment of high blood cholesterol in adults (Adult Treatment Panel III). JAMA 2001;285:2486–97.
18. Hebert PR, Pfeffer MA, Hennekens CH. Use of statins and aspirin to reduce cardiovascular disease. J Cardiovasc Pharmacol Ther 2002;7:77–80.
19. Hennekens CH, Sacks F, Tonkin A, et al. Additive benefits of pravastatin and aspirin to decrease risks of cardiovascular disease: randomized and observational comparisons of secondary prevention trials and their meta-analysis. Arch Intern Med 2004;164:40–4.

20. Berry SM, Berry DA, Natarajan K, et al. Bayesian survival analysis with non-proportional hazards: meta-analysis of combination of pravastatin-aspirin. J Am Stat Assoc 2004;99:36–44.
21. Sandler RS, Halabi S, Baron JA, et al. A randomized trial of aspirin to prevent colorectal adenomas in patients with previous colorectal cancer. N Engl J Med 2003;348:883–90.
22. Baron JA, Cole BF, Sandler RS, et al. A randomized trial of aspirin to prevent colorectal adenomas. N Engl J Med 2003;348:891–9.
23. Bibbins-Domingo K, on behalf of the U.S. Preventive Services Task Force. Aspirin use for the primary prevention of cardiovascular disease and colorectal cancer: U.S. preventive services task force recommendation statement. Ann Intern Med 2016;164:836–45.
24. Collins R, Reith C, Emberson J, et al. Interpretation of the evidence for the efficacy and safety of statin therapy. Lancet 2016;388(10059):2532–61.
25. Cholesterol Treatment Trialists' (CTT) Collaboration, Baigent C, Keech A, Kearny PM, et al. Efficacy and safety of cholesterol-lowering treatment: prospective meta-analysis of data from 90 056 participants in 14 randomised trials of statins. Lancet 2005;366(9493):1267–78.
26. Cholesterol Treatment Trialists (CTT) Collaboration, Kearney PM, Blackwell L, Collins R, et al. Efficacy of cholesterol-lowering in 18,686 people with diabetes in 14 randomised trials of statins: a meta-analysis. Lancet 2008;371:117–25.
27. Cholesterol Treatment Trialists' (CTT) Collaboration, Baigent C, Blackwell L, Emberson J, et al. Efficacy and safety of more intensive lowering of LDL cholesterol: a meta-analysis of data from 170,000 participants in 26 randomized trials. Lancet 2010;376:1670–81.
28. Cholesterol Treatment Trialists (CTT) Collaboration, Mihaylova B, Emberson J, Blackwell L, et al. The effects of lowering LDL cholesterol with statin therapy in people at low risk of vascular disease: meta-analysis of individual data from 27 randomised trials. Lancet 2012;380:581–90.
29. Cholesterol Treatment Trialists' (CTT) Collaboration, Fulcher J, O'Connell R, Voysey M, et al. Efficacy and safety of LDL-lowering therapy among men and women: meta-analysis of individual data from 174 000 participants in 27 randomised trials. Lancet 2015;385:1397–405.
30. Hennekens CH, Lieberman E, Rubenstein M, et al. Lipid Modification in the Treatment and Prevention of Cardiovascular Diseases: Emerging clinical and public health challenges. In: Watson RR, editor. Handbook of cholesterol. Urbana (IL): AOCS Press; 2016. p. 155–81 [Chapter 9].
31. Ridker PM, Danielson E, Fonseca FA, et al. Rosuvastatin to prevent vascular events in men and women with elevated C-reactive protein. N Engl J Med 2008;359:2195–207.
32. Ridker PM, Cushman M, Stampfer MJ, et al. Inflammation, aspirin, and the risk of cardiovascular disease in apparently healthy men. N Engl J Med 1997;336:973–9.
33. Hennekens CH. Statin-induced myopathy: hypothesis about randomized evidence and clinical impressions. Am J Med 2009;122(1):4–5.
34. Stone NJ, Robinson JG, Lichtenstein AH, et al. American College of Cardiology/American Heart Association Task Force on Practice Guidelines 2013 ACC/AHA guideline on the treatment of blood cholesterol to reduce atherosclerotic cardiovascular risk in adults: a report of the American College of Cardiology/American Heart Association Task Force on Practice Guidelines. Circulation 2014;129(25 Suppl 2):S1–45.

35. Pung M, Robishaw J, Pfeffer M, et al. Prescription of statins to women poses new clinical challenges. Am J Med 2018;131(10):1139–40.
36. Hennekens CH, Pfeffer M, Newcomer J, et al. Treatment of diabetes mellitus: the urgent need for multifactorial interventions. Am J Manag Care 2014;20(5):357–9.
37. Hennekens CH, D'Agostino R Sr. Global risk assessment for cardiovascular disease and astute clinical judgement. Eur Heart J 2003;8:12–3.
38. Hennekens CH, Sherling DH. Prescription of statins to the elderly: clinical and public health challenges. Ger Med 2016;9:34.
39. Hennekens CH, Pfeffer M. Guidelines and guidance in lipid modification. Trends Cardiovasc Med 2015;25:348–50.
40. Gitin A, Pfeffer MA, Hennekens CH. Editorial commentary: the lower the LDL the better-but how and how much? Trends Cardiovasc Med 2018;28(5):355–6.

Prevention of Hypertension Related to Cardiovascular Disease

Parvathi Perumareddi, DO

KEYWORDS

- Hypertension • Blood pressure • Risk factors • Lifestyle modifications • Prevention
- Cardiovascular disease

KEY POINTS

- Hypertension is among the most common conditions encountered in primary care practices.
- As blood pressure increases, associated cardiovascular risk also increases.
- Risk factors may be nonmodifiable, such as age, race, and family history, or modifiable, associated with environment or lifestyle.
- Guidelines have become more stringent in an effort to prevent cardiovascular disease (CVD), which will likely result in larger prevalence of diagnosed hypertension.
- Modifiable risk factors can be improved by lifestyle modifications including healthier diet, lower dietary sodium intake, maintaining a normal body mass index or weight, limiting alcohol intake, and exercise resulting in reduced blood pressure and CVD risk.

INTRODUCTION

Hypertension is among the most common conditions encountered by primary care physicians. An estimated 1 in 3 adults in the United States has hypertension.[1]

Blood pressure is maintained or regulated by several factors, including intravascular volume, cardiac output, peripheral vascular resistance, and the elasticity of the blood vessels. There is also an autoregulatory mechanism in place, the renin-angiotensin system, which involves the kidneys; however, if there is a disruption in this mechanism, the result is elevated blood pressure, often leading to hypertension.[2]

Although frequently asymptomatic, it is an important modifiable risk factor for cardiovascular disease (CVD), which remains the leading cause of death both in the United States and globally.

It is known that, as blood pressure increases, there is a clinically significant association with risk of CVDs,[3] arteriosclerotic disease, and other diseases, such as congestive heart failure and cerebrovascular disease.

Disclosure Statement: The author has nothing to disclose.
Charles E. Schmidt College of Medicine, Florida Atlantic University, 777 Glades Road, ME-104, Room 213, Boca Raton, FL 33431, USA
E-mail address: pperumar@health.fau.edu

Prim Care Clin Office Pract 46 (2019) 27–39
https://doi.org/10.1016/j.pop.2018.10.005
0095-4543/19/© 2018 Elsevier Inc. All rights reserved.

Despite advances in pharmacotherapy and increased knowledge of the disease state, high blood pressure is often inadequately controlled. The poor control can be attributed to lack of awareness, costly medicines, and barriers to treatment, as well as the asymptomatic nature of the disease until late in its course.

CLINICAL DESCRIPTION OF THE DISEASE

There are many factors that influence the progression and toward hypertension, including genetic and environmental. The exact mechanism of the genetic influence remains unknown; however, inadequate volume regulation, enhanced vasoconstriction, and changes in the arterial wall (eg, increased resistance and decreased luminal diameter), are all known to lead to increased blood pressure.[2,4,5]

Hypertension is divided into 2 categories: primary (or essential) hypertension and secondary hypertension. Primary hypertension is defined as a chronic elevation in blood pressure without a known cause. Both genetic and environmental factors play in a role in the development of primary hypertension, which makes up approximately 90% to 95% of cases.[2]

Secondary hypertension is an elevation in blood pressure due to a known cause and constitutes the remaining 5% to 10% of cases. Of equal importance is the known inevitability that blood pressure increases with age, such that most adults develop hypertension by the age of 70 years. Therefore, it is important to be diligent in addressing blood pressure at earlier ages to prevent the progression to hypertension, as well as to be aggressive with treatment of those who develop it.

In the past several years, the level at which a provider diagnoses hypertension has been spotlighted and is based on guidelines by various entities, with even more focus on the thresholds for treatment and goal blood pressure levels.

The Joint National Committee (JNC) defined hypertension in their seventh report (JNC 7) as a blood pressure of greater than or equal to 140/90 mm Hg on at least 2 different occasions, separated by at least 1 week.[6] The JNC later convened to update their 2003 JNC 7 guidelines and released their latest report in 2014.

JNC 8 recommendations were written on evidence-based data obtained through a detailed literature review. The previous guidelines were based on studies with various designs, whereas the JNC 8 guidelines were based solely on randomized controlled trials (RCTs).[7]

Although the definition of blood pressure in terms of level was not addressed, the thresholds for treatment were. In JNC 8, a major revision was the proposal that individuals in the general population aged 60 years or older could be treated starting at a systolic blood pressure (SBP) of 150 mm Hg or diastolic blood pressure (DBP) of 90 mm Hg as evidenced that there was no outcome advantage to setting and reaching lower goals. It was taken into consideration that there may be many patients in this age range who had already achieved a blood pressure of less than 140 mm Hg, thus the recommendation followed that there was no need to take action by reducing their medications to increase their blood pressure to 150 mm Hg. Interestingly, there were members of the panel who disagreed with this goal and recommended that the previous JNC 7 guidelines be followed in terms of blood pressure reduction for all populations, regardless of age, to the lower level of 140/90 mm Hg. It was, however, unanimously decided that more research is needed to determine the ideal goal SBP for these patients.[7]

Shortly after the JNC 8 guidelines were issued, the results from the Sprint Research Group were released. The Systolic Blood Pressure Intervention Trial (SPRINT) was a landmark multicenter trial involving more than 9000 subjects enrolled in an RCT to determine whether lower target SBP would result in a reduction in cardiovascular events.

Criteria for the study included SBP greater than or equal to 130 mm Hg and an increased cardiovascular risk, excluding diabetes. The targets that were investigated were SBPs of 140 mm Hg (standard) versus 120 mm Hg (intensive arm). The study was halted early based on findings that there were significantly lower rates of cardiovascular events, both fatal and nonfatal, in the intensive study group. This included myocardial infarction, cerebrovascular accident, acute decompensated heart failure, and death. These findings were also confirmed in elderly individuals aged 75 years and older.[8]

The limitations found within the trial included the percentage of serious adverse events (eg, hypotension, syncope, falls, bradycardia) that occurred in the intensive treatment arm; therefore, the investigators issued a caveat that caution should be exercised if treating the elderly to these new goal levels.[8] Another factor unique to this study was the method used to measure the blood pressures: Subjects were kept in a quiet room alone for at least 10 minutes, after which their blood pressure was measured at least 3 times and averaged.[8] This brought to light a discussion on the inconsistencies in blood pressure measurement methods, as well as the improbability that this practice is performed outside of a standardized and controlled trial, meaning blood pressures in real populations are taken in different environments and with different methods than those measured with carefully controlled procedures within a study.

In 2017, almost 2 years after the release of SPRINT, the American College of Cardiology/American Heart Association Task Force (ACC/AHA) released guidelines for the prevention, detection, evaluation, and management of high blood pressure in adults. The recommendations by the ACC/AHA were based on reviews and meta-analyses when possible and were focused on not only treatment thresholds but also a redefinition of the level at which hypertension is diagnosed. However, the definition of normal blood pressure remained unchanged. The rationale for reclassifying the upper end of prehypertension was due to the thought that there is about a 2-fold increase in CVD risk in this blood pressure range, as well as the benefit found in recent RCTs that a blood pressure less than 130 mm Hg is more desirable in terms of outcomes. Of note, the goal blood pressure for individuals with known CVD or a CVD equivalent remains less than or equal to 130/80 mm Hg.[9]

In considering the most recent guideline definitions of hypertension by ACC/AHA, it is important to note that the prevalence of hypertension is expected to increase considerably, necessitating an increase in the number of individuals requiring treatment.

Despite there not being a consensus on the level of blood pressure that constitutes hypertension or what threshold and goal to treat to, all the committees did reinforce recommendations of the need for lifestyle modifications as a first step in addressing high blood pressure. They also all shared the recommendation that, when there was a need for an antihypertensive, specific classes of antihypertensives should be chosen based on comorbidities.

The stages of hypertension as defined by the various organizations are shown in **Table 1**.

CLASSIFICATION OF BLOOD PRESSURE
Epidemiology

According to data obtained from the National Health and Nutrition Examination Survey from 2015 to 2016 (using the JNC 7 definition of hypertension), the prevalence of hypertension was found to be 29%. This increased with age, such that the highest

Table 1
Stages of hypertension as defined by organization guidelines

Organization	Classification	SBP (mm Hg)	DBP (mm Hg)
ACC/AHA	Normal blood pressure (BP)	≤120	≤80
	Elevated BP	120–129	≤80
	Stage 1 hypertension (HTN)	130–139	80–89
	Stage 2 HTN	≥140	≥90
JNC 7 or JNC 8, 2014	Normal BP	≤120	≤80
	Pre-HTN	120–139	80–89
	Stage 1 HTN	140–159	90–99
	Stage 2 HTN	≥160	≥100

Data from Refs.[6,7,9]

percentage occurred in the population aged 60 years and older. Of note, men had and continue to have a higher prevalence of hypertension until age 60 years, at which time women have higher rates.[1]

Regarding racial or origin stratification, the prevalence was highest among black persons, followed by white persons, Asians, and Hispanics (**Figs. 1** and **2**).[1]

Unfortunately for hypertensive adults, only 48.3% or so were labeled as having controlled hypertension, using JNC 7 criteria.[1] This trend continues, illustrating the lack of adequate control of hypertension.

Secondary hypertension occurs much less frequently than primary hypertension and is associated with another causal disease states or exogenous causes (see

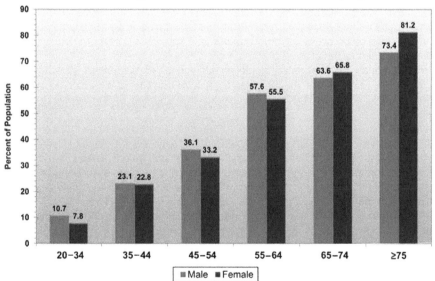

Fig. 1. Prevalence of Hypertension in the United States by age and sex. (*Data from* Fryar CD, Ostchega Y, Hales CM, et al. Hypertension prevalence and control among adults: United States, 2015-2016. NCHS data brief, no 289. Hyattsville (MD); National Center for Health Statistics: 2017.)

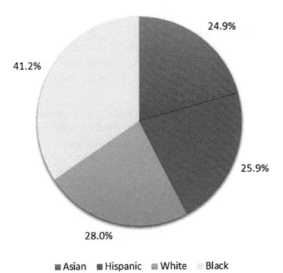

24.9%

41.2%

25.9%

28.0%

■ Asian   ■ Hispanic   ■ White   ■ Black

Fig. 2. Prevalence of hypertension by race or origin. (*Data from* Fryar CD, Ostchega Y, Hales CM, et al. Hypertension prevalence and control among adults: United States, 2015-2016. NCHS data brief, no 289. Hyattsville (MD); National Center for Health Statistics: 2017.)

previous discussion). A high index of suspicion for secondary hypertension and its causes should arise in cases of patients with resistant hypertension despite aggressive antihypertensive therapy or those with significant hypokalemia.

Other reasons to suspect secondary hypertension include specific symptoms native to various disorders. For example, if a patient develops abrupt onset hypertension or if their hypertension becomes difficult to manage, the provider should suspect some type of renovascular disease. These patients may present with arterial bruits, either an abdominal bruit, or in another location, such as the femoral artery or the carotid artery.[9] Primary aldosteronism is typically suspected in hypertensive patients who have hypokalemia. Symptoms such as muscle weakness or muscle cramps may be associated with primary hyperaldosteronism. Obstructive Sleep Apnea (OSA) is commonly associated with resistant hypertension and snoring. Although there is a small occurrence of hypertension due to drugs or alcohol, this can be minimized by being conscious of and limiting the potential for secondary hypertension with judicious use of nonsteroidal antiinflammatory drugs (NSAIDs), oral contraceptive pills (OCPs), decongestants, herbal agents, and other medicines. Symptoms such as tachycardia, fine tremor, and sweating may suggest secondary hypertension secondary to use of cocaine and ephedrine,[9] thus patients should be counseled to avoid these.

Although caffeine use is very common and generally benign, there can be elevation in blood pressure with caffeine intake.[9] This may also manifest with tachycardia or palpitations; therefore, if these symptoms are present, the patient's caffeine consumption should be ascertained.

The following are potential causes of secondary hypertension in order of prevalence[9]:

- OSA (25%–50%)
- Renal disease (5%–34%)
  - Chronic renal disease
  - Renal artery stenosis

- ○ Polycystic kidney disease
- Primary aldosteronism (8%–20%)
- Alcohol, drugs, or exogenous substances (2%–4%)
  - ○ Ethanol, cocaine, methamphetamine, nicotine, licorice, erythropoietin, OCPs, decongestants, NSAIDs, herbals (eg, ephedra, ma huang), some psychiatric medications, and steroids.

For women taking Oral contraceptive pills (OCPs) who develop resultant hypertension (approximately 5%), it typically resolves within 6 months of discontinuation of OCPs (5A). Exogenous steroids are linked with elevated blood pressure primarily through intravascular volume expansion. NSAIDs exert their effect by an increase in sodium retention, as well as by inhibition of the vasodilatory effects of prostaglandins and increased production of vasoconstricting factors such as endothelin-1.

Studies have demonstrated OSA to be an independent risk factor for the development of hypertension, exclusive of obesity. Almost 50% of individuals with OSA have hypertension. During apneic spells, there is an increase in sympathetic activity such that blood pressure rises.[10] These persons are known to have a higher associated cardiovascular mortality.

More uncommon causes of secondary hypertension include[2]

- Pheochromocytoma
- Adrenocortical dysfunction (Cushing syndrome, congenital adrenal hyperplasia)
- Hypothyroidism or hyperthyroidism
- Coarctation of the aorta
- Primary hyperparathyroidism
- Acromegaly
- Collagen vascular disease or vasculitis.

Common risk factors associated with primary hypertension are listed in **Table 2**.

NONMODIFIABLE RISK FACTORS
Family History

Hypertension is definitively observed in individuals with a family history; however, the exact genetic influence remains unknown.[2]

Age

An increase in blood pressure occurs as vasculature becomes less elastic, which occurs as an age-related situation (see previous discussion). It is primarily SBP that

Table 2 Common risk factors associated with primary hypertension	
Genetic	**Environmental**
Family History	Obesity
Age	Diet
Race	Sodium intake
Insulin resistance	Alcohol consumption

Data from Chobanian AV, Bakris GL, Black HR, et al. The seventh report of the Joint National Committee on prevention, detection, evaluation, and treatment of high blood pressure: the JNC 7 report. JAMA 2003;290(2):197.

increases with age, such that most people older than the age of 70 years have hypertension.

Race

Hypertension is both more common and more severe in African Americans.[1] The cause is unclear; however, some research suggests that African Americans may have relatively lower renin levels, as well as salt sensitivity.

Obesity Related to Insulin Resistance

It has been long established that overweight or obese individuals are more likely to develop hypertension. Some of this is due to genetic predisposition to lower insulin sensitivity; however, recent focus has been on the effect of the actual fat distribution in obese patients with their predetermined insulin resistance. In other words, all individuals are born with a certain level of insulin sensitivity; however, in those who develop obesity, the insulin resistance is greatly increased. Studies have demonstrated that a more important factor is the location of the adiposity; specifically, a large waist-to-hip ratio is a greater indication of visceral fat.[11] This is often referred to as central obesity (abdominal fat).

The risks are less with lower body obesity in which the fat deposits are located in the legs and buttocks. The former is a problem because visceral fat leads to insulin resistance and multiple metabolic derangements, which result in metabolic syndrome leading to significantly higher chance of CVD. The exact relationship between the neuroendocrine effects of the adiposity on hypertension is unknown; however, it is thought that the adipocytes produce the hormone leptin, which may have an effect on metabolism and appetite, as well as on the hypothalamus, thus increasing blood pressure via activation of the sympathetic nervous system.[11]

The remainder of this article highlights the modifiable risk factors associated with primary hypertension.

SCREENING

Certain populations are at a greater risk for hypertension (see previous discussion). The recommendations for screening are shown in **Table 3**.

Although the timing for hypertension screening is important, so is the method used. Recent guidelines have suggested a departure from diagnosing blood pressure in clinics or office visits due to the inaccuracy of measurements in the office setting because this is often based on user variability during auscultation of Korotkoff sounds, as well as other factors. It has become important to factor in the expected variation in blood pressure in a 24-hour day per normal physiology.

Recently, position for measurement was tested and it was found more desirable to take blood pressure in the seated position with both feet on the floor.[15]

Recent focus has been on allowing the patient to have blood pressure taken outside the office by either home-based pressure monitoring (HBPM) or ambulatory blood pressure monitoring (ABPM). These methods can detect nondippers; that is, individuals whose blood pressure does not physiologically fall nocturnally.[16] This is important because nondippers are known to be more at risk for CVD. White coat hypertension, which has been historically associated with falsely elevated blood pressures, can also be detected through HBPM.

Both HBPM and ABPM have been associated with lower and more accurate blood pressure readings, thus they have become the recommended methods as better predictors of CVD risk than office readings.[9]

Table 3 Screening recommendations			
Organization	Population	Measurement	Interval
USPSTF	≥18 y general population	HBPM or ABPM	Every 3–5 y
	High-risk population		Annually
JNC7	≥18 y with BP <120/80 mm Hg		Recheck 2 y
	≥18 y with BP 120 139/80–89 mm Hg		Annually
ACOG	Females ≥13 y		Annually with well visit
AAP	≥3 y general population		Annually
	high risk population		Every visit

Abbreviations: AAP, American Academy of Pediatrics; ACOG, American College of Obstetricians and Gynecologists; USPSTF, United States Preventive Services Task Force.
Data from Refs.[12–14]

Lifestyle Modifications for Prevention and Treatment of Hypertension

Although risk factors should be addressed regularly, so should the possible therapeutic lifestyle changes in an effort to aim for prevention of hypertension. However, when an individual belongs in the category of having elevated blood pressure or prehypertension, depending on which guideline is followed, it is recommended to begin treatment by initiating a trial of lifestyle modifications. It should be noted, however, that this should be for a prescribed period before reevaluating. Most of the guidelines recommend a trial of 3 to 6 months[6,7,9] before commencing antihypertensive therapy. When the decision is made that antihypertensive therapy should begin, the importance of lifestyle modification maintenance should be stressed.

Importantly, blood pressure reduction is observed in both hypertensive patients and normotensive persons who maintain lifestyle modifications.

Weight loss

The aim is to reduce body weight to that which achieves a normal body mass index (BMI); however, it has been shown that even modest reductions in weight result in a linear relationship with blood pressure reduction. Approximately 1 mm Hg reduction in blood pressure may be achieved for every 2.3 lb of weight loss.[9] In fact, even in normotensive individuals, weight loss results in lower blood pressure.[16] Patients should be educated on the importance of monitoring not only weight but also measurement of waist circumference and BMI (charts or a BMI calculator can be useful). With the advent of technology on smartphones, there are a vast array of tools and telephone applications that can aid patients with tracking their weight, and as well as ways to reduce weight and waist circumference (ideal is <40 in for men and <35 in for women). Food journals for tracking calories are often helpful in weight loss efforts. Some patients may find that support groups are useful in terms of accountability. Physicians may consider using a team-based approach with dieticians, nutritionists, and exercise personnel, which may reinforce and/or complement patient education and compliance.

Healthy diet

In large trials, the Dietary Approaches to Stop Hypertension (DASH) diet promoted by the National, Heart, Lung, and Blood Institute has been shown to result in significant reductions in blood pressure independent of weight loss.[17] This diet is rich in fruits, vegetables, nuts, fish, poultry, and grains; has reduced saturated fat and cholesterol intake; uses low-fat dairy; and has minimal amounts of sugars and red meat.[18]

Along with the aforementioned general dietary food groups, patients can be taught how to review and interpret nutritional labels to be aware of their daily intake and the properties of several macronutrients (fats, proteins, carbohydrates), as well as calorie counting.

Reduction in sodium intake

The recommended limit of dietary sodium intake per ACC/AHA guidelines is less than 1500 mg/d or 1.5 g/d; however, it has been shown that even modest reductions in sodium from high to medium to low result in lower blood pressures (ref/cite). It is important to ensure that patients be made aware of the sources of dietary sodium because many assume that merely not adding salt at the table or during food preparation and cooking is considered adequate. They should be counseled that many food items are high in sodium (ie, canned foods, cheeses, breads, and many processed foods). Most food items are now required to carry labels of their nutritional content. If counseled appropriately, patients can know their specific sodium intake merely by monitoring labels for their dietary intake. Of note, combining the DASH diet and sodium reduction has been proven to provide even more benefit in lowering blood pressure than either intervention alone.[19]

Potassium supplementation

It has been suggested that inadequate levels of potassium may contribute to hypertension; therefore, it is recommended that diet be modified such that potassium is supplemented this way.[20] The recommended amount is 3.5 to 5 g/d.[9]

Alcohol consumption

An early study from the Oakland–San Francisco Kaiser Permanente Medical Care Program showed a link between consistent alcohol intake and increased blood pressure. In this study of 84,000 individuals, it was revealed that the regular intake of 3 or more drinks per day resulted in an increased risk for hypertension.[21] SBP was found to be affected more than DBP; however, the exact mechanism is unclear.

The maximum recommended amounts of alcohol are less than or equal to 2 drinks daily for men and less than or equal to 1 drink daily for women, corresponding to a 12 oz beer, 5 oz wine, or 1.5 oz of distilled spirits.[9]

Physical activity

The most commonly prescribed physical activity or exercise is aerobic. Most guidelines provided advocate specific amounts of cardiovascular exercise, which are 150 minutes per week or 30–40 minutes most days of the week.[22] Patients should be counseled to monitor their heart rate and maintain it to between 65% and 75% of their maximum, which is calculated based on the formula of 220 beats per minute minus age. It is important to stress that the effect of aerobic exercise is limited, so performing the entire amount of exercise on a weekend as opposed to throughout the week has not been shown to confer the same benefit. Also shown to be helpful is providing tailored aerobic exercise to fit the needs of each patient, while paying attention to their physical limitations, their access to equipment, and their interests. For example, patients with arthritis or joint problems can often exercise in the pool without added stress and pain to their joints. For others, engaging in organized sports provides aerobic benefits that are enjoyable.

There is also evidence that weight or resistance training reduces blood pressure. Significance reductions in resting blood pressure have been observed in as few as 4 to 5 weeks of isometric resistance training,[23] thus this is a helpful adjunct to aerobic exercise.

To obtain adherence to exercise, it is helpful to provide a structured or prescribed exercise program in terms of type, quantity, and frequency because people are more likely to follow and maintain these activities.

Stress reduction

Psychosocial stress is a ubiquitous lifestyle factor that contributes to increased blood pressure. Studies have demonstrated that chronic stress and hypertension are linked to subsequent cardiac disease, which is mediated via continuous overactivation of the sympathetic nervous system. A meta-analysis found that transcendental meditation supported blood pressure reduction.[24]

There is disagreement about whether biofeedback is helpful, although some studies report that it can provide benefits.[25]

No recommendations have been made; however, stress reduction tips may be suggested.

Tobacco cessation

There is a strong association between smoking and CVD. Smoking immediately causes excessive stimulation of the sympathetic nervous system, resulting in increased myocardial oxygen demand, thus resulting in increased heart rate, blood pressure, and contractility.[25] Patients should be educated and counseled at every visit regarding tobacco use, as well as assessed for readiness to quit. Cessation tools should be offered.

Outcomes for Patients and Complications

The prevention of hypertension is an important step in reducing the overall burden of CVD because it has been shown in clinical trials that there is a decrease in mortality with reduction in blood pressure. Incidence of myocardial infarction, congestive heart failure, and cerebrovascular disease is lowered significantly (**Fig. 3**).[6]

Despite advances in pharmacotherapy and increased knowledge, there remains a large population with hypertension, which is often inadequately controlled. Poor control may be attributed to lack of patient awareness, costly medicines, and barriers to treatment, as well as the asymptomatic nature of the disease until late in its course.

Hypertension is thought to cause CVD through several mechanisms. It hastens atherogenesis and causes degenerative changes in the vessel wall, such as thickening and proliferation of vascular smooth muscle cells. Ultimately, this can lead to serious complications such as cerebrovascular hemorrhage and aortic dissection. Because the endothelium modulates the growth of the vascular smooth muscle, endothelial dysfunction, such as in hypertension or atherosclerotic CVD, can cause arterial or arteriolar wall thickening and reduction of luminal diameter. These changes alter the vessels elasticity and ability to accommodate changes in blood pressure.[2]

Further, hypertension is thought to exhibit its deleterious effects by causing oxidative stress in the arterial wall. This may result in activation of an inflammatory response that, if coupled with dyslipidemia, leads to atheroma formation.[2]

The SBP is representative of the amount of blood (stroke volume) pumped from the heart, as well as the rate and elastic compliance of major arteries (ie, aorta). The walls of the vessels are elastic until late in life when they become more rigid, resulting in an

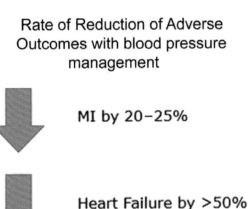

Rate of Reduction of Adverse Outcomes with blood pressure management

MI by 20–25%

Heart Failure by >50%

CVA by 35–40%

Fig. 3. Rate of Reduction of Adverse Outcomes with blood pressure management. CVA, cerebrovascular accident; MI, myocardial infarction. (*Data from* Chobanian AV, Bakris GL, Black HR, et al. The seventh report of the Joint National Committee on prevention, detection, evaluation, and treatment of high blood pressure: the JNC 7 report. JAMA 2003;290(2):197.)

increased SBP, an anticipated occurrence as age progresses past the seventh decade.

An increase in SBP (afterload) causes the left ventricle to work harder by increasing the pressure against which the heart must pump as it ejects blood. As afterload increases, the wall of the left ventricle becomes larger and thicker (ie, hypertrophies) despite this compensatory mechanism.[26] Left ventricular hypertrophy becomes a risk factor, not only for congestive heart failure but also for dysrhythmias, coronary artery disease, and sudden death.[2]

The multiple pathologic conditions caused by high blood pressure result in various forms of CVD; therefore, it is important to prevent these underlying causes.

SUMMARY

Hypertension is a disease state with a strong link to CVD with resultant devastating effects. It is often asymptomatic, which makes screening vital. Current trends reveal hypertension is occurring at younger ages and within a larger percentage of the population, and this number will increase should lower thresholds for diagnosis be used.

Because of the high prevalence and clear pathologic burden of hypertension and its profound ramifications, it is important to not only use early screening and detection but also preventative measures. Primary care providers see hypertensive patients frequently and the vital impact of prevention can be achieved with collaboration between the provider and patient with education, counseling, and a shared partnership in decision-making.

> **Box 1**
> **Strategies for the prevention of hypertension**
>
> - Screening of blood pressure at recommended intervals
> - Use of home-based pressure monitoring or ambulatory blood pressure monitoring for more accurate readings of blood pressure
> - Patient education of risk factors for development of hypertension
> - Prevention and/or treatment of obesity (especially waist circumference)
> - Physical activity or exercise
> - Dietary Approaches to Stop Hypertension (DASH) diet
> - Low-sodium diet
> - Incorporation of potassium-rich diet
> - Limited alcohol consumption
> - Avoidance of or cessation of smoking or tobacco products
> - Avoidance of illicit drugs (eg, cocaine)
> - Use caution with over-the-counter medications and herbal preparations and drug–drug interactions

Risk factors should be addressed regularly but education should also be provided early in life and continued longitudinally to ensure adherence and avoid long-term morbidity (**Box 1**). It is imperative that primary care providers, who often encounter patients not only during disease but also for well visits, are vigilant in efforts to prevent and reduce hypertension. This includes removing barriers for the patient. The ideal way to accomplish this is through a patient-centered model in which the patient is educated on prevention of hypertension, its potential complications, and the strategies to avoid this disease; is involved in self-management; and shares in medical decision-making.

REFERENCES

1. Fryar CD, Ostchega Y, Hales CM, et al. Hypertension prevalence and control among adults: United States, 2015-2016. NCHS data brief, no 289. Hyattsville (MD): National Center for Health Statistics; 2017.
2. Kumar V, Abbas AK, Aster JC. Robbins and Cotran pathologic basis of disease. 9th edition. Philadelphia: Elsevier/Saunders; 2015.
3. Liszka H, Mainous A, King D, et al. Prehypertension and cardiovascular morbidity. Ann Fam Med 2005;3:294–9.
4. Alexander W. Hypertension and the pathogenesis of atherosclerosis oxidative stress and the mediation of arterial inflammatory response: a new perspective. Hypertension 1995;25:155–61.
5. Staessen J, Wang J, Bianchi G, et al. Essential hypertension. Lancet 2003;361: 1629–41.
6. Chobanian AV, Bakris GL, Black HR, et al. The seventh report of the Joint National Committee on prevention, detection, evaluation, and treatment of high blood pressure: the JNC 7 report. JAMA 2003;290(2):197.
7. James PA, Oparil S, Carter BL, et al. 2014 evidence-based guideline for the management of high blood pressure in adults: report from the panel members

appointed to the Eighth Joint National Committee (JNC 8). JAMA 2014;311(5): 507–20.

8. The Sprint Research Group. A randomized trial of intensive versus standard blood-pressure control. N Engl J Med 2015;373:2103–16.

9. ACC/AHA/AAPA/ABC/ACPM/AGS/APhA/ASH/ASPC/NMA/PCNA guideline for the prevention, detection, evaluation, and management of high blood pressure in adults: a report of the American College of Cardiology/American Heart Association Task Force on clinical practice guidelines. J Am Coll Cardiol 2017. [Epub ahead of print].

10. Alexander M. Hypertension: practice essentials, background, and physiology. Theheart.org. Medscape 2018.

11. Mathieu P. Visceral obesity the link among inflammation, hypertension and cardiovascular disease. Hypertension 2009;53:577–84.

12. United States Preventative Services Task Force. High Blood Pressure in Adults: Screening. October 2015.

13. American College of Obstetrics and Gynecology. Well-Woman Recommendations. Available at: https://www.acog.org/About-ACOG/ACOG-Departments/Annual-Womens-Health-Care/Well-Woman-Recommendations. Accessed December, 2018.

14. AFP Editors. Screening and management of high BP in children and adolescents: an updated guideline from the AAP. Am Fam Physician 2018;97(8):543–4.

15. Morcos R, Carter K, Castro F. Getting the hypertension Dx right: patient positioning matters. J Fam Pract 2018;67(4):199–207.

16. Bacon S, Sherwood A, Hindliter A, et al. Effects of exercise, diet and weight loss on high blood pressure. Sports Med 2004;34(5):307–16.

17. Dickinson H, Mason J, Nicolson D, et al. Lifestyle interventions to reduce raised blood pressure: a systematic review of randomized controlled trials. J Hypertens 2006;24:215–33.

18. Sacks F, Svetkey L, Vollmer W, et al. Effects on blood pressure of reduced dietary sodium and the Dietary Approaches to Stop Hypertension (DASH) diet. N Eng J Med 2001;344(1):3–10.

19. Langan R, Jones K. Common questions about the initial management of hypertension. Am Fam Physician 2015;91(3):172–7.

20. Sacks F, Willett W, Smith A, et al. Effect on blood pressure of potassium, calcium and magnesium in women with low habitual intake. Hypertension 1998;31:131–8.

21. Klatsky A, Freidman GD, Siegelaub AB. Alcohol consumption and blood pressure. N Engl J Med 1977;296:1194–200.

22. Cornelissen V, Smart N. Exercise training for blood pressure: a systematic review and meta-analysis. J Am Heart Assoc 2013;2:e004473.

23. Millar P, McGowan C. Evidence for the role of isometric exercise training in reducing blood pressure: potential mechanisms and future directions. Sports Med 2014;44:345–56.

24. Rainforth M, Schneider R, Nidich S, et al. Stress reduction programs in patients with elevated blood pressure: a systematic review and meta-analysis. Curr Hypertens Rep 2007;9(6):520–8.

25. Rupal O, Garcellano M. Nonpharmacologic management of hypertension: what works? Am Fam Physician 2015;91(11):772–6.

26. Alpert M, Lavie C, Agrawal H, et al. Obesity and heart failure: epidemiology, pathophysiology, clinical manifestations and management. Transl Res 2014;164(4): 345–435.

The Screening and Prevention of Diabetes Mellitus

Lisa C. Martinez, MD*, Dawn Sherling, MD, Allison Holley, MD

KEYWORDS

- Diabetes mellitus • Screening • Prevention • Complications • Metformin
- Hemoglobin A1C

KEY POINTS

- Diabetes mellitus is characterized by metabolic diseases that result in hyperglycemia.
- Type 2 diabetes (T2D) mellitus makes up most diabetes diagnoses, with at least 90% of patients having this type.
- Patients with T2D mellitus have gradual hyperglycemia and often do not recognize the classic symptoms of hyperglycemia because of the indolent onset of the disease; however, patients can develop microvascular and macrovascular complications before diagnosis, making screening for this disease crucial to prevent complications.
- Although it is important for clinicians to be vigilant for all forms of diabetes mellitus, owing to the overwhelming prevalence of T2D mellitus in primary care practices, this article focuses on the screening for and the complications of T2D mellitus.

CLINICAL DESCRIPTION

For primary care providers, type 2 diabetes (T2D) mellitus is among the most common diseases seen in practice. Diabetes mellitus is characterized by metabolic diseases that result in hyperglycemia. It is typically the result of defects in insulin secretion, insulin sensitivity or action, or both. Diabetes mellitus can be categorized into 4 classifications:

- Type 1 diabetes (T1D) mellitus
- T2D mellitus
- Gestational diabetes mellitus (GDM)

Disclosure: The authors have nothing to disclose.
Department of Integrated Medical Sciences, Charles E. Schmidt College of Medicine, Florida Atlantic University, 777 Glades Road, 71-140, Boca Raton, FL 33498, USA
* Corresponding author.
E-mail address: lmartinez@health.fau.edu

Prim Care Clin Office Pract 46 (2019) 41–52
https://doi.org/10.1016/j.pop.2018.10.006
0095-4543/19/© 2018 Elsevier Inc. All rights reserved.

primarycare.theclinics.com

- Diabetes mellitus due to other causes, such as diseases of the exocrine pancreas or drug-induced diabetes mellitus.

T2D mellitus makes up most diabetes mellitus diagnoses, with at least 90% of patients having this type.[1] T2D mellitus has a multifaceted pathophysiology that includes insulin resistance and beta cell dysfunction.[2] Patients with this type of diabetes mellitus have gradual hyperglycemia and often do not recognize the classic symptoms of hyperglycemia because of the indolent onset of the disease. However, despite the lack of symptoms, these patients can be developing microvascular and macrovascular complications before diagnosis, making screening for this disease crucial to prevent complications.[3]

T1D is the result of insulin deficiency due to destruction of pancreatic beta cells, resulting in insulin deficiency. This type of diabetes mellitus affects between 4% and 6% of all diabetics, and is typically immune-mediated with autoantibodies to islet cells, insulin, glutamic acid decarboxylase, protein tyrosine phosphatase (ICA512 or IA2A), and zinc transporter protein 8.[4,5] The presentation of T1D is typically much more acute than that of T2D mellitus. Children usually present with ketoacidosis as the first manifestation, whereas adults can have a more indolent presentation that can often mimic that of T2D mellitus.[4] GDM describes diabetes mellitus diagnosed during the second or third trimester of pregnancy,[3] which can be associated with adverse perinatal outcome, including increased risk of Cesarean section and macrosomia.[6,7] Although many women will revert to euglycemia after their pregnancy, those with GDM have at least a 7-fold increased risk for developing diabetes mellitus later in life, making screening of this population very important.[8]

In addition to those who are diagnosed with diabetes mellitus, many patients are classified as having intermediate hyperglycemia or a high-risk state for developing diabetes mellitus, sometimes referred to as prediabetes mellitus. Similar to patients with T2D mellitus, these patients have insulin resistance and beta cell dysfunction but their levels of hyperglycemia do not reach the threshold for diagnosis of diabetes mellitus. Patients in this intermediate hyperglycemic state have a markedly increased risk of developing diabetes mellitus, with 5% to 10% of patients in this state progressing to overt diabetes mellitus annually.[9]

Although it is important for clinicians to be vigilant for all forms of diabetes mellitus, due to the overwhelming prevalence of T2D mellitus in primary care practices, this article focuses on the screening for and the complications of T2D mellitus.

EPIDEMIOLOGY

Using information from the National Health and Nutrition Examination Survey (NHANES) data, it is estimated that diabetes mellitus affects 9.4% to 12.3% of the US population, with 7.2 million Americans (23.8%) unaware of their diagnosis.[1,10] These numbers have been steadily increasing since 1988.[10] There are an estimated 1.5 million new cases of diabetes mellitus diagnosed in adults annually, with more than 90% attributed to T2D mellitus.[1,2] Furthermore, approximately 33.9% (84 million) of adults 18 years or older and 48.3% of adults 65 years or older have intermediate hyperglycemia, or prediabetes mellitus.[1] Diabetes mellitus also confers a tremendous amount of morbidity and mortality, with more than 7 million hospital discharges and 14 million emergency department visits annually listing diabetes mellitus as a diagnosis.[1] It is currently listed as the seventh leading cause of death in the United States.[9]

As previously described, GDM and prediabetes mellitus are both risk factors for the subsequent development of T2D mellitus. However, there are many other risk factors with which a clinician needs to be familiar. Heredity plays a role: patients have a 2.4-fold increase if a first-degree family history is present, and an even higher risk if both maternal and paternal history of diabetes mellitus is present.[2] Ethnicity also plays a role: data from the Nurses' Health Study shows increased risk in Asians, Hispanics, and African Americans compared with whites.[11,12] Obesity seems to play an even larger role than either heredity or ethnicity: the increase in prevalence of diabetes mellitus from 1976 to 2010 in women was seemingly completely attributable to the increase in body mass index (BMI) over the same time period. In men, BMI has also been noted to be the greatest contributor the increased prevalence of T2D mellitus.[10] Although the NHANES data were unable to link physical activity to risk for diabetes mellitus, a study of Swedish military service participants showed that low aerobic capacity and muscle strength tripled the risk for T2D mellitus, even among those with a normal BMI.[13] Other risk factors for the development of diabetes mellitus are listed in **Box 1**.

SCREENING FOR TYPE 2 DIABETES MELLITUS

A crucial component in the prevention of T2D mellitus is screening those at risk, recognizing prediabetes mellitus, and promptly educating the at-risk patient on lifestyle changes and preventive measures. Several different organizations have guidelines on which patients should be screened, how often, and the cut-off laboratory values for prediabetes mellitus (**Table 1**). For the purposes of this article, only guidelines pertaining to nonpregnant adults are discussed. Additional guidelines for pregnant adults, as well as adolescents and children, are not included.

The US Preventive Services Task Force (USPSTF) recommends screening overweight or obese adults who are between 40 and 70 years old. Patients who are high-risk, such as those who have a family history of diabetes mellitus or a personal history of GDM, or who are members of high-risk ethnic groups, could be screened at an earlier age or lower BMI.[19]

The American Diabetes Association (ADA) recommends screening overweight or obese adults who have at least 1 risk factor for diabetes mellitus starting at age 45 years and subsequently every 3 years thereafter if results are normal.[3] The ADA recommends using any of the following for screening: fasting plasma glucose, 2-hour

---

Box 1
Risk factors for development of type 2 diabetes mellitus

- Prediabetes mellitus (impaired fasting glucose, impaired glucose tolerance, or hemoglobin A1c >5.7%)
- First-degree relative with diabetes mellitus[2]
- Ethnicity (Hispanic, Asian, and African-American)[11,12]
- Obesity[10]
- Sedentary lifestyle[13]
- Smoking[14]
- History of GDM[8]
- Polycystic ovarian syndrome[15]
- Hypertension[16]
- Cardiovascular disease[17]
- Metabolic syndrome.[18]

Table 1
Organization guidelines for diabetes mellitus screening

Organization	Patients That Should be Screened	Frequency
US Preventive Services Task Force	• Overweight or obese adults 40–70 y of age	Every 3 y

American Diabetes Association	• All adults >45 y
	• All adults who are overweight or obese and have 1 additional risk factor:
	  ○ Physical inactivity
	  ○ First-degree relative with diabetes mellitus
	  ○ High-risk race or ethnicity
	  ○ Hypertension ≥140/90 (or on treatment)
	  ○ History of cardiovascular disease
	  ○ High-density lipoprotein cholesterol <35 mg/dL and/or triglycerides >250 mg/dL Women with polycystic ovarian syndrome
	  ○ Women with polycystic ovarian syndrome
	  ○ Other clinical conditions associated with insulin resistance (ie, severe obesity, acanthosis nigricans)
	• Adults with prediabetes mellitus
	• Women who were diagnosed with GDM
		At least every 3 y, more frequently depending on results

American Association of Clinical Endocrinologists	Same as ADA guidelines with following additions: • Patients on antipsychotic therapy • Patients with chronic glucocorticoid exposure • Sleep disorders in the presence of glucose intolerance	Every 3 y, and annually for patients with ≥2 risk factors

plasma glucose after administration of 75 g oral glucose tolerance test, or hemoglobin A1c.[3] To diagnose prediabetes mellitus, any among the following results are required: fasting plasma glucose of 100 to 125 mg/dL, or 2-hour plasma glucose after 75 g oral glucose tolerance test of 140 to 199 mg/dL, or hemoglobin A1c of 5.7% to 6.4%.[3] To diagnose diabetes mellitus, any of the following can be used: fasting plasma glucose of greater than or equal to 126 mg/dL, or random plasma glucose of greater than or equal to 200 mg/dL, or a 2-hour plasma glucose after a 75 g oral glucose tolerance test of greater than or equal to 200 mg/dL, or a hemoglobin A1c of 6.5% or more.[3] If any of the aforementioned tests are positive, repeat testing using any of the modalities is recommended, performed on a different day, to confirm the diagnosis of diabetes mellitus.[3]

The American Association of Clinical Endocrinologists (AACE) has similar guidelines for diagnosing prediabetes mellitus, with the exception of lowering the needed value of hemoglobin A1c to establish the diagnosis of prediabetes mellitus to 5.5%. AACE guidelines also advise that the diagnosis of prediabetes mellitus should be confirmed with repeat testing on a different day.[20] Importantly, AACE considers hemoglobin A1c for diagnosis of diabetes mellitus as a secondary test, which needs to be confirmed with fasting plasma glucose levels (see later discussion of the rationale).[20]

A diabetes mellitus risk factor worksheet has been made available on the ADA's Web site at diabetes.org. This can be provided to patients in the waiting room or at an office visit, to further assist clinicians in assessing who to screen.

PREVENTION OF TYPE 2 DIABETES MELLITUS

T2D mellitus has affected the world at epidemic levels, unmatched by any other chronic illness. It is has, therefore, become incumbent on medical professionals to assist patients in preventing diabetes mellitus and the complications associated with this disease. Several studies have been done that show the promise of both lifestyle interventions and medication in the prevention of diabetes mellitus.

The Diabetes Prevention Program (DPP) spanned from 1996 to 2001 and had 3 arms: the intensive lifestyle intervention arm, the metformin arm, and the placebo arm.[21] The DPP was a randomized controlled trial and included 27 centers with 3234 participants, all of whom were overweight with prediabetes mellitus and included a high proportion (45%) of minority groups because these groups are disproportionately affected by diabetes mellitus.[21] The lifestyle intervention arm included diet, exercise (consisting of at least 150 minutes of brisk walking or similar activity per week), 16 structured educational sessions, a life coach, additional follow-up education and feedback, and a toolbox of strategies to encourage long-term commitment to the lifestyle changes.[21] These interventions resulted in a 58% decrease in the development of diabetes mellitus when compared with placebo.[21]

During the metformin arm of the DPP, patients were assigned to standard lifestyle changes that included recommendations to follow the food guide pyramid, use a National Cholesterol Education Program Step 1 diet, lose weight, and increase their physical activity, along with the administration of metformin 850 mg taken orally, titrated up to twice daily as permitted by gastrointestinal side effects.[22-24] Those receiving metformin had a 31% lower incidence of diabetes mellitus when compared with those receiving placebo, although not as great a reduction as those in the lifestyle intervention group.[21]

The DPP Outcomes Study (DPPOS) was a follow up of the DPP and evaluated the long-term benefits of lifestyle intervention and metformin on preventing diabetes mellitus and preventing microvascular disease, which was defined as nephropathy, retinopathy, and neuropathy.[25] The DPPOS analyzed 2776 of the participants from DPP using an intention-to-treat analysis from 2002 to 2014. In the lifestyle intervention arm, the rate of developing diabetes mellitus was reduced by 27%, and in the metformin arm by 18%. The development of microvascular complications was not significantly different between the arms.[25] However, in those who did not develop diabetes mellitus, their microvascular complication rate was 28% less than those who did develop diabetes mellitus.[25] These findings should encourage medical providers to work hard with patients to prevent diabetes mellitus. To facilitate this, the

Medicare program is slated to begin to reimburse and cover the costs of CDC-recognized DPP lifestyle programs in April 2018.[26]

Several other studies have investigated the effect of lifestyle changes on development of T2D mellitus. Three important studies are the Da Qing Impaired Glucose Tolerance (IGT) and Diabetes Study, the 20-year follow-up study of the Da Qing study, and the Finnish Diabetes Prevention Study. The Da Qing IGT and Diabetes Study was performed starting in 1986 and studied 577 subjects in China with IGT, randomizing them into 1 of 4 groups: a control group, a diet-only group, an exercise-only group, and a diet plus exercise group.[27] The subjects were followed every 2 years for a total of 6 years. At the end of the 6 years, the investigators examined the proportion of subjects whose laboratory results had progressed from IGT to T2D mellitus.[27] They found that, compared with the control group in which 67.7% had advanced to diabetes mellitus, only 43.8% had developed diabetes mellitus in the diet group, 41.1% had developed diabetes mellitus in the exercise group, and 46% had developed diabetes mellitus in the diet plus exercise group, demonstrating that diet and/or exercise can play a role in decreasing the likelihood of developing diabetes mellitus.[27]

In 2006, a 20-year follow-up study was done on the original cohort in the Da Qing Study, in which varying levels of follow-up data were available on 568 of the participants.[28] Development of macrovascular and microvascular complications, and all-cause mortality, were assessed.[28] The lifestyle intervention groups were combined and taken together had a 51% reduction in developing diabetes mellitus when compared with the control group during the 6 years of the original Da Qing study and a 43% reduction in developing diabetes mellitus during the follow-up 20 years later.[28] However, no statistically significant differences were found in the rates of complications, cardiovascular mortality, or all-cause mortality, which the investigators speculated could have been due to the limited statistical power of the study.[28]

The Finnish Diabetes Prevention Study enrolled a total of 522 participants in Finland from 1993 to 1998 with the stated goal of 3 years of follow-up for each of the enrollees. However, there was early termination of the study in 2000 secondary to the high rates of reduction of diabetes mellitus in the intervention group.[29] Study subjects in this trial were overweight or obese, aged 40 to 64 years old, and had IGT. Among the primary goals that distinguished the Finnish study was its attempt to use lifestyle interventions that were practical and feasible for primary care physicians in the treatment of patients at risk for developing diabetes mellitus.[29] The control group participants were given only general advice regarding diet and exercise in a 30 minute to 1 hour individual or group session. The lifestyle intervention group participants were given individualized instruction with a nutritionist for 30 minutes to 1 hour in 7 sessions in the first year of the study and then every 3 months subsequently.[29] The intensive lifestyle group was also given strict criteria for diet and exercise, including the goal of 0.5 to 1 kg of weight loss per week maximum, a total weight loss goal of 5% or greater, at least 30 minutes of moderate intensity exercise daily, fat in the diet of less than 30% total energy, saturated fat of less than 10% total energy, and at least 15 g of fiber for every 1000 kcal.[29] Other supportive measures for the lifestyle intervention group included the availability of group sessions, special guest lectures, field trips to supermarkets, cooking classes, periodic phone calls, and food logs, which were submitted quarterly.[29] Ultimately, the intensive lifestyle intervention group had a 58% reduction in the development of diabetes mellitus when compared with the control group.[29]

The aforementioned studies demonstrated that diabetes mellitus can be prevented in a clinical setting, whereas the Prevent-DM trial was done to study the effectiveness of preventing diabetes mellitus in a community setting.[30] Prevent-DM was a randomized controlled trial of 92 Latina women from 2013 to 2015. The 3 arms of the trial were similar to the DPP, with an intensive lifestyle treatment arm, metformin 850 mg taken orally twice daily, and a control group that received standard care.[30] Patients had their weight, blood pressure, waist circumference, and laboratory tests (fasting glucose, insulin, lipids, and hemoglobin A1C) measured at the beginning of the study and then again at 12 months.[30] The Prevent-DM intensive lifestyle intervention arm had mean weight loss of 5% compared with 1.1% in the metformin arm and 0.9% in the standard-care arm.[30] The intensive lifestyle intervention arm also had a decrease in waist circumference when compared with the standard-care arm and a small improvement in hemoglobin A1C when compared with both the metformin arm and the standard-care arm.[30]

There have also been several studies examining the effects that specific diets have on the prevention of T2D mellitus. As previously noted, studies have included dietary modifications in their lifestyle treatment arms. In addition, there have been additional studies demonstrating that low carbohydrate diets, diets with low glycemic index foods, high-fiber diets, diets high in monounsaturated and polyunsaturated fats, and diets with high linoleic acid, can all decrease the risk of developing diabetes mellitus.[31–34]

In 2017, an analysis regarding omega-6 fatty acid biomarkers was done to determine if the incidence of diabetes mellitus was affected by dietary consumption of omega-6 polyunsaturated fatty acids (mainly linoleic acid and arachidonic acid).[34] This was a pooled analysis of 20 different prospective cohort studies done previously across the world that included adult subjects who did not have diabetes mellitus at baseline.[34] This study found that linoleic acid consumption seemed to reduce the risk of developing diabetes mellitus, whereas arachidonic acid did not.[34] Of note, the study did not include US participants and the source of linoleic acid (ie, deep fried processed foods vs olive oil or nuts) which may matter in the finding of the reduction of diabetes mellitus incidence.[35] Some investigators think that increasing dietary linoleic acid may in fact decrease the incidence of diabetes mellitus if coming from the right sources, including full-fat dairy products, nuts, olive oil, and legumes, rather than other unhealthy oils or buttery type spreads.[35]

OUTCOMES AND COMPLICATIONS

With more than 100 million Americans diagnosed as diabetic or prediabetic,[36] it becomes critical that the outcomes of screening and prevention endeavors are examined. Along with blood pressure and lipid control, lowering blood glucose has been shown to prevent or slow the onset of microvascular complications. Intensive lifestyle interventions have been shown to delay the onset of diabetes mellitus by as many as 14 years.[28]

Although the long-term benefits are clear, the short-term benefits of screening have been difficult to ascertain, with mortality and cardiovascular benefits most likely accruing 23 to 30 years after diagnosis.[37] There is stronger evidence for reduction in microvascular complications when diabetics are brought under control sooner.[38] These microvascular complications include retinopathy, nephropathy, and diabetic neuropathies. These produce significant morbidity in patients, leading to loss of vision, loss of kidney function, impaired mobility, difficulties with cognition, and inability to work, increasing not only the quality of life costs to the patient but financial costs to society as a whole.[39] Therefore, at the time of diagnosis of T2D mellitus additional screening should be done for concurrent conditions for which patients with T2D mellitus are at high risk, including[38]

- Dyslipidemia: lipid panel
- Nephropathy: serum creatinine and urine microalbumin
- Retinopathy: ophthalmology referral
- Neuropathy: clinical examination of feet, including skin integrity, pedal pulses, monofilament testing, vibration sense, and ankle reflexes.

As the number of people with diabetes mellitus increases, the costs associated with the care of both diagnosed and undiagnosed Americans with diabetes mellitus has been estimated at more than $100 billion in direct costs and is projected to triple to more than $300 billion over the next 25 years.[40] With an eye to both the cost and morbidity associated with diabetes mellitus, there has been a broad effort aimed at prevention of this disease.

As previously noted, although the DPP was highly effective, the cost was estimated at $2700 per participant.[41] Community-based programs such as the YMCA's DPP have attempted to achieve similar results by encouraging a regimen of lifestyle changes in participants at an average cost of $400 per participant.[42] The investigators of this trial estimated that medical savings due to prevention of diabetes in participants would result in a net benefit to payers in as little as 3 years' time.[42]

According to the USPSTF, there is transient anxiety but no long-term psychological harm that can be expected from discovery of an elevated blood glucose. There is little to no downside in instituting lifestyle modifications, the first-line treatment for an elevated blood glucose, though there can be harms produced by the medications used in treatment.[43]

Patients aged 65 years or older have been shown to have a reduced incidence of T2D mellitus with diagnosis of the disease increasing up until this point and then leveling off. Combined with the data that suggest that benefits of early diagnosis and treatment are more clearly seen after approximately 2 decades, there is some justification for the USPSTF recommendation to stop screening older adults.[38,44,45] However, it is conceivable that older adults will have a random blood glucose done in the course of work-up or monitoring of other illnesses and many of them, incidentally, will be found to have elevations in their blood glucose. How aggressively to manage these patients has been evolving, with current guidelines suggesting that higher hemoglobin A1c targets, or perhaps no hemoglobin A1c target, may be desirable and may help to avoid polypharmacy and hypoglycemia in this more medically fragile population.[44,45] A more detailed discussion of the treatment of T2D mellitus is outside of the scope of this article.

Taking into consideration that many patients who are diagnosed with diabetes mellitus or prediabetes mellitus have comorbidities and may take many other medications, whatever their age, it is vital that the diagnoses resulting from screening efforts are accurate.

The adoption of hemoglobin A1C as a screening tool for T2D and prediabetes mellitus was not without initial controversy. Indeed, as previously noted, AACE guidelines recommend that a fasting plasma glucose test be used to confirm the diagnosis of prediabetes mellitus if the initial screening test was a positive hemoglobin A1C alone.[20] There are many ways that the hemoglobin A1C measurement may be prone to error. Point-of-care machines for hemoglobin A1C, which are being used more widely, open the possibility for occasional unreliable results.[46] There are also ethnic variations in hemoglobin A1c testing, with African Americans being more prone to false-positive tests and white persons prone to more false-negative tests.[47,48] Levels

Box 2	
Causes of changes in hemoglobin A1c levels	
Causes of Increased A1c	**Causes of Decreased A1c**
• Iron deficiency	• Erythropoietin
• B12 deficiency	• Iron
• Alcoholism	• Vitamin B12
• Chronic renal failure	• Chronic liver disease
• Splenectomy	• Antiretroviral drugs
• Chronic opioid use	• Ribavirin
• Hemoglobinopathies	• Dapsone
	• Hypertriglyceridemia
	• Hemoglobinopathies

Data from Gallagher EJ, Le Roith D, Bloomgarden Z. Review of hemoglobin A(1c) in the management of diabetes. J Diabetes 2009;1(1):9–17.

of hemoglobin A1C increase as the age of the red blood cell increases.[48] In other words, the longer the red blood cell survives in the circulation, the higher the A1c, whereas the shorter time the red blood cell is allowed to circulate, the lower the hemoglobin A1c, even for equivalent measures of blood glucose.

It has also been noted that certain medications can affect hemoglobin A1c measurements.[49] Thus, clinical judgment must be exercised when interpreting this now widely used screening measure to avoid confusion and possible diagnostic and management errors. Hemoglobin A1c is perhaps a more reliable measure of blood glucose variation within an individual, although caution should be exercised in comparing the hemoglobin A1c of a patient to another patient, whose differences in hemoglobin A1c may not be reflective of differences in blood glucose levels but rather in their red blood cell life span, comorbidities, and other genetic factors (**Box 2**). In the aggregate, the harms from screening are quite small, whereas the morbidity, mortality, and cost benefits that may accrue from prevention and early diagnosis of this devastating disease are demonstrably many times greater.

REFERENCES

1. Centers for Disease Control and Prevention. National Diabetes Statistics Report, 2017. Atlanta, GA: Centers for Disease Control and Prevention, US Department of Health and Human Services; 2017.

2. Stumvoll M, Goldstein B, van Haeften T. Type 2 diabetes: principles of pathogenesis and therapy. Lancet 2005;364(9467):1333–46.

3. American Diabetes Association. Classification and diagnosis of Diabetes: Standards of Medical Care in Diabetes-2018. Diabetes Care 2018;41(S1):S13–27.

4. Chang J, Kirkman MS, Laffel L, et al. Type 1 diabetes through the life span: a position statement of the American Diabetes Association. Diabetes Care 2014;37: 2034–54.

5. Menke A, Orchard TJ, Imperatore G, et al. The prevalence of type 1 diabetes in the United States. Epidemiology 2013;24(5):773–4.

6. Metzger B, Gabbe SG, Persson B, et al. International Association of Diabetes and Pregnancy Study Groups Recommendations on the Diagnosis and Classification of Hyperglycemia in Pregnancy. Diabetes Care 2010;33(3):676–82.

7. Kampmann U, Madsen L, Skajaa G, et al. Gestational diabetes: a clinical update. World J Diabetes 2015;6(8):1065–72.

8. Bellamy L, Casas JP, Hingorani AD, et al. Type 2 diabetes mellitus after gestational diabetes: a systematic review and meta-analysis. Lancet 2009;373:1773–9.

9. Tabak A, Herder C, Rathmann W, et al. Prediabetes: a high-risk state for diabetes development. Lancet 2012;379:2279–90.

10. Menke A, Rust K, Fradkin J, et al. Associations between trends in race/ethnicity, aging, and body mass index with diabetes prevalence in the United States: a series of cross-sectional studies. Ann Intern Med 2014;161:328–35.

11. Menke A, Casagrande S, Geiss L. Prevalence of and trends in diabetes among adults in the United States, 1988-2012. JAMA 2015;314(1):1021–9.

12. Shai I, Jiang R, Manson J, et al. Ethnicity, obesity and risk of type 2 diabetes in women: a 20 year follow-up study. Diabetes Care 2006;29(7):1585–90.

13. Crump C, Sundquist J, Winkleby M, et al. Physical fitness among Swedish military conscripts and long-term risk for type 2 diabetes mellitus: a cohort study. Ann Intern Med 2016;164(9):577–84.

14. Willi C, Bodenmann P, Ghali WA, et al. Active smoking and the risk of type 2 diabetes: a systematic review and meta-analysis. JAMA 2007;298(22):2654–64.

15. Ehrmann D, Barnes R, Rosenfield R, et al. Prevalence of impaired glucose tolerance and diabetes in women with polycystic ovary syndrome. Diabetes Care 1999;22(1):141–6.

16. Conen D, Ridker P, Mora A, et al. Blood pressure and risk of developing type 2 diabetes mellitus: the women's health study. Eur Heart J 2007;28(23):2937.

17. Mozaffarian D, Masfisi R, Levantesi G, et al. Incidence of new-onset diabetes and impaired fasting glucose in patients with recent myocardial infarction and the effect of clinical and lifestyle risk factors. Lancet 2007;370:667–75.

18. Ford E, Li C, Sattar N. Metabolic syndrome and incident diabetes: current state of the evidence. Diabetes Care 2008;31(9):1898–904.

19. *Final Recommendation Statement: Abnormal Blood Glucose and Type 2 Diabetes Mellitus: Screening.* U.S. Preventive Services Task Force; 2018. Available at: https://www.uspreventiveservicestaskforce.org/Page/Document/Recommendation StatementFinal/screening-for-abnormal-blood-glucose-and-type-2-diabete. Accessed February 21, 2018.

20. American Association of Clinical Endocrinologists Board of Directors, American College of Endocrinologists Board of Trustees. American Association of Clinical Endocrinologists/American College of Endocrinology statement on the use of hemoglobin A1c for the diagnosis of diabetes. Endocr Pract 2010;16:155–6. Available at: http://outpatient.aace.com/type-2-diabetes/diagnosis-of-type2-diabetes-mellitus. Accessed February 21, 2018.

21. Diabetes Prevention Program (DPP) Research Group. The Diabetes Prevention Program (DPP): description of lifestyle intervention. Diabetes Care 2002;25(12): 2165–71.

22. Diabetes Prevention Program (DPP) Research Group. Reduction in the Incidence of Type 2 Diabetes with Lifestyle Intervention or Metformin. N Engl J Med 2002; 345(6):393–403.

23. United States Department of Agriculture. The food guide pyramid. Washington, DC: Department of Agriculture, Center for Nutrition Policy and Promotion; 1996 (Home and Garden Bulletin no. 252).

24. Step by Step: eating to lower your high blood cholesterol. Bethesda (MD): National Heart, Lung, and Blood Institute Information Center; 1987.

25. Diabetes Prevention Research Group. Long-term effects of lifestyle intervention or metformin on diabetes development and microvascular complications over 15-year followup: the Diabetes Prevention Program Outcomes Study. Lancet Diabetes Endocrinol 2015;3:866–75.
26. Delahanty LM. Weight loss in the prevention and treatment of diabetes. Prev Med 2017;104:120–3.
27. Pan XR, Li GW, Hu YH, et al. Effects of diet and exercise in preventing NIDDM in people with impaired glucose tolerance: the Da Qing IGT and Diabetes Study. Diabetes Care 1997;20:537–44.
28. Li G, Zhang P, Wang J, et al. The long-term effect of lifestyle intervention to prevent diabetes in the China Da Qing Diabetes Prevention Study: a 20-year follow-up study. Lancet 2008;371(9626):1783–9.
29. Tuomilehto J, Lindstrom J, Eriksson JG, et al. Prevention of type 2 diabetes mellitus by changes in lifestyle among subjects with impaired glucose tolerance. N Engl J Med 2001;344:1343–50.
30. O'Brien M, Perez A, Scanlan AB, et al. PREVENT-DM comparative effectiveness trial of lifestyle intervention and metformin. Am J Prev Med 2017;52(6):788–97.
31. Salmeron J, Ascherio A, Rimm EB, et al. Dietary fiber, glycemic load and risk of NIDDM in men. Diabetes Care 1997;20(4):545–50.
32. Salmeron J, Hu FB, Manson JE, et al. Dietary fat intake and risk of type 2 diabetes in women. Am J Clin Nutr 2001;73:1019–26.
33. Salmeron J, Manson JE, Stampfer MJ, et al. Dietary fiber, glycemic load, and risk of NIDDM in women. JAMA 1997;277(6):472–7.
34. Wu J, Marklund M, Tintle N, et al. Omega-6 fatty acid biomarkers and incident type 2 diabetes: pooled analysis of individual-level data for 39740 adults from 20 prospective cohort studies. Lancet Diabetes Endocrinol 2017;5:965–74.
35. Henderson G, Crofts C, Schofield G. Linoleic acid and diabetes prevention. Lancet Diabetes Endocrinol 2018;6:12–3.
36. 2011–2014 National Health and Nutrition Examination Survey (NHANES), National Center for Health Statistics, Centers for Disease Control and Prevention.
37. Pippitt K, Li M, Gurgle HE. Diabetes mellitus: screening and diagnosis. Am Fam Physician 2016;93(2):103–9.
38. Handelsman Y, Bloomgarden ZT, Grunberger G, et al. American Association of Clinical Endocrinologists and American College of Endocrinology—clinical practice guidelines for developing a diabetes mellitus comprehensive care plan—2015. Endocr Pract 2015;21(suppl 1):1–87.
39. Valencia WM, Florez H. How to prevent the microvascular complications of type 2 diabetes beyond glucose control. BMJ 2017;356:i6505.
40. Huang ES, Basu A, O'Grady M, et al. Projecting the future diabetes population size and related costs for the U.S. Diabetes Care 2009;32(12):2225–9.
41. Herman WH, Brandle M, Zhang P, et al. Costs associated with the primary prevention of type 2 diabetes mellitus in the Diabetes Prevention Program. Diabetes Care 2003;26(1):36–47.
42. Vojta D, Koehler TB, Longjohn M, et al. A coordinated national model for diabetes prevention: linking health systems to an evidence-based community program. Am J Prev Med 2013;44(4 Suppl 4):S301–6.
43. Abnormal Blood Glucose and Type 2 Diabetes Mellitus: Screening - US Preventive Services Task Force: Final Recommendation Statement. Available at: https://www.uspreventiveservicestaskforce.org/Page/Document/RecommendationStatementFinal/screening-for-abnormal-blood-glucose-and-type-2-diabetes. Accessed March 8, 2018.

44. Kirkman SM, Briscoe VJ, Clark N, et al. Diabetes in older adults. Diabetes Care 2012;35(12):2650–64.

45. Qaseem A, Wilt TJ, Kansagara D, et al. Hemoglobin A1c targets for glycemic control with pharmacologic therapy for nonpregnant adults with type 2 diabetes mellitus: a guidance statement update from the American College of Physicians. Ann Intern Med 2018;168(8):569–76.

46. Malkani S, Mordes JP. Implications of using hemoglobin A1C for diagnosing diabetes mellitus. Am J Med 2011;124(5):395–401.

47. Olson DE, Rhee MK, Herrick K, et al. Screening for diabetes and prediabetes with proposed A1c-based diagnostic criteria. Diabetes Care 2010;33(10):2184–9.

48. Cohen RM, Haggerty S, Herman WH. HbA1c for the diagnosis of diabetes and prediabetes: is it time for a mid-course correction? J Clin Endocrinol Metab 2010;95(12):5203–6.

49. Gallagher EJ, Le Roith D, Bloomgarden Z. Review of hemoglobin A(1c) in the management of diabetes. J Diabetes 2009;1(1):9–17.

Immunizations

Benjamin B. Wilde, DO*, David J. Park, DO

KEYWORDS

- Immunization • Vaccine • Prevention • Public health • Shots • Health maintenance

KEY POINTS

- Vaccination is among the most effective preventative health measures to date.
- All recommended vaccines should be administered together at the appropriately scheduled time.
- Vaccines may be administered at intervals longer than the recommendation schedule without significant loss of immunity; however, they should not be administered on an accelerated schedule.
- True contraindications to vaccinations are limited to individuals with a history of anaphylaxis, encephalopathy, severe combined immunodeficiency syndrome, and intussusception (rotavirus).

INTRODUCTION

Vaccination has been observed to be among the most effective preventative health measures in the modern era, second only to clean water.[1] Certain vaccines, such as the *Haemophilus influenza* type b (Hib) vaccine, protect an individual before exposure to the disease; others, such as rabies, hepatitis A and B, and varicella vaccines, can be protective following exposure. Vaccines are classified as inactivated; live attenuated; toxoid; or subunit, recombinant, polysaccharide, and conjugate vaccines. A list of common vaccines from each classification is shown in **Table 1**.[2,3]

Live-attenuated vaccines contain a weakened form of the microorganism that can still replicate and induce an immune response but should not cause disease. Responses to this type of vaccine are very similar to that of a mild natural infection. Therefore, usually 1 dose is sufficient to produce immunity. A second dose, the so-called booster, is often recommended to further enhance the response to the vaccine. These vaccines are the most prone to adverse reactions and, in individuals with immunodeficiency, even harmful sequelae.

Inactivated vaccines contain components of the virus or bacteria that have been inactivated or killed with heat and/or chemicals. These organisms can no longer

Disclosure Statement: The authors have nothing to disclose.
Department of Primary Care, Rocky Vista University College of Osteopathic Medicine–Southern Utah, 255 East Center Street, Ivins, UT 84738, USA
* Corresponding author.
E-mail address: bwilde@rvu.edu

Prim Care Clin Office Pract 46 (2019) 53–68
https://doi.org/10.1016/j.pop.2018.10.007

Table 1 Vaccine types and examples of each		
Type of Vaccine	**Examples**	
Live Attenuated	Intranasal influenza Measles Mumps Polio (oral) Rotavirus Rubella	Shingles Smallpox Varicella Yellow fever Zoster
Inactivated	Hepatitis A Influenza (intramuscular)	Polio (intramuscular) Rabies
Toxoid	Diphtheria	Tetanus
Subunit, Recombinant, Polysaccharide, and Conjugate	Hib Hepatitis B Human papillomavirus	Pertussis Pneumococcal Meningococcal

Data from Hamborsky J, Kroger A, Wolfe S. Epidemiology and prevention of vaccine-preventable diseases. 13th edition. Washington, DC: Public Health Foundation; 2015.

replicate or cause disease. Because the organism has been significantly changed from the structure of the disease-causing organism, it takes multiple doses to sufficiently prime and stimulate the immune response.

Toxoid vaccines use an attenuated form of a toxin to induce immunity, not the toxin-producing organism itself. Periodic boosters are required for toxoid vaccines.

Subunit, recombinant, polysaccharide, and conjugate vaccines contain specific parts of an organism to induce an immune response.

EPIDEMIOLOGY

Vaccinations have been proven to effectively lower overall mortality, diminish disease sequelae, and lead to milder disease severity in the event of an occurrence.[4] It is estimated that vaccines prevent 6 million deaths worldwide annually.[4] They protect not only those immunized but also reduce the incidence of disease among the nonimmunized individuals of a community. Additional documented benefits of vaccination include substantial decreases in both direct and indirect health care costs, a decline in antibiotic resistance, extended life expectancy, safer global travel and mobility, enhanced protection against bioterrorism, promotion of economic growth (especially in developing countries), and decreased disparity between racial and socioeconomic groups.[4]

According to the Centers for Disease Control and Prevention (CDC) so-called Pink Book, since the advent of immunizations, the world has seen a sharp decline in what are now considered vaccine-preventable diseases.[2] Most dramatically, when comparing the twentieth century annual morbidity in the United States with its current (2017) morbidity, smallpox and diphtheria dropped 100%. Morbidity for conditions such as polio, measles, rubella, and Hib dropped greater than 99%. Mumps and pertussis morbidity dropped 97% and 92%, respectively. In the twentieth century, these conditions combined would have amounted to more than 1 million patients afflicted annually in the United States alone. In contrast, these same conditions in 2017 resulted in only 21,623 cases, merely 0.02% of total annual instances of the previous century.[5]

GENERAL RECOMMENDATIONS
Timing Intervals

Increasing the interval between doses of a multidose vaccine does not diminish the effectiveness of the vaccine (after the series has been completed).[6(p13)] Studies have shown no difference in the final titer of a vaccine series with extended intervals. Therefore, it is not necessary to restart a vaccination series or give additional doses to achieve a protective immune response when the recommended interval schedule is delayed.

The opposite, however, is not true. Shortening the intervals of a multidose vaccine can interfere with the desired antibody response. Accelerated vaccination schedules should be avoided. Vaccinations are considered valid when given up to 4 days before the recommended interval.

The immune response to some vaccines can wane over time. Additional booster doses are indicated at defined intervals. This is most common for tetanus, pertussis, and diphtheria vaccines.

Administration

All recommended vaccinations should be administered at the same visit when possible. Such an approach has not been shown to decrease antibody responses to the different vaccines or to increase the incidence of adverse events. Simultaneous administration of both parenteral and oral vaccinations, be it live attenuated or inactivated, has not been shown to have negative affect on vaccine efficacy. If live vaccines are not administered together, they should be spaced by at least 4 weeks.

Combination vaccinations are generally preferred compared with single-component vaccines when possible. This can simplify the immunization process significantly by reducing the number of injections, facilitating vaccine availability, reducing cost, and improving patient coverage. One exception to this is the measles, mumps, rubella (MMR)–varicella (MMRV) combination vaccine. This combination can increase the risk of febrile seizures in children and should not be used in children younger than 47 months of age.[7] When given before that age, the 2 vaccines should be administered separately.

Most immunizations are administered intramuscularly. Exceptions include the oral rotavirus vaccine (RV), the intradermal or intranasal influenza vaccine (the intranasal vaccine is not currently recommended as part of the schedule), and the subcutaneous MMRV-containing vaccines. Pneumococcal polysaccharide 23 (PPSV23) and inactivated poliovirus vaccines can be given intramuscularly or subcutaneously.

Adverse Reactions

Any problematic effect caused by a vaccine can be considered an adverse reaction or side effect. Such adverse reactions should be closely monitored and documented, irrespective of whether it is a true adverse reaction or merely a coincidental event. Adverse reactions are categorized as local, systemic, or allergic. Up to 80% of vaccinations will cause localized pain, swelling, and redness, and are usually self-limited. Systemic reactions include fever, malaise, and/or headache. They occur less frequently in inactivated vaccines. Systemic reactions in response to a live attenuated vaccine will typically have a 3-day to 21-day incubation period, and can result in symptoms similar to a mild form of the natural disease. All clinically significant adverse reactions should be reported to the US Vaccine Adverse Event Reporting System.[8]

Contraindications

It is important to understand when a vaccination is contraindicated or special precautions should be taken. When an individual is at increased risk for an adverse reaction associated with serious harm, certain vaccines should not be given. These contraindications may be permanent or temporary. There are 3 contraindications that are considered permanent:

1. Severe allergic reaction (anaphylaxis) to a vaccine component or following a prior dose
2. Encephalopathy occurring within 7 days of pertussis vaccination without other identifiable cause
3. Rotavirus vaccine is contraindicated in individuals with severe combined immunodeficiency (SCID) or a history of intussusception.

Some vaccination providers incorrectly define additional conditions as contraindications. These special considerations include current illness, current or recent antimicrobial therapy, recent disease exposure or convalescence, pregnancy, breastfeeding, preterm birth, allergy to products not present in the vaccine, an allergy that is not anaphylactic, family history of adverse events, tuberculin skin testing (TST), multiple vaccines, or presence of an immunosuppressed person in the household.[6] Current antiviral drug treatment is considered a precaution to varicella vaccination.[9]

SPECIAL CONSIDERATIONS

Some conditions that warrant deviation from the standard immunization schedule are listed in the following sections. For a full list, see **Box 1**.[6]

Allergy

A vaccine is contraindicated when a patient has demonstrated an anaphylactic allergic response to any vaccine component. The most common allergic response is to egg protein, which has been used as a medium for preparing the yellow fever and influenza vaccines.

Pregnancy

A pregnant patient should not receive live vaccines. Although only smallpox vaccine has proven to cause fetal injury, the theoretic concern of a live vaccine causing injury to the fetus has resulted in this standard of care. Inactivated vaccines, including influenza, are safe to administer. One exception, human papillomavirus (HPV), has not received full approval for use in pregnancy due to lack of data currently.

Preterm Infant

Vaccinations should be administered according to chronologic age of the infant. If the infant weighs less than 2000 g, the first hepatitis B dose administered before discharge from the hospital does not count toward the series, which is subsequently started at 1 month of age.

Breastfeeding

A breast-feeding mother should receive all vaccines except yellow fever. A breast-feeding infant should receive all routine childhood vaccines. Breast-feeding has not been found to extend maternal-infant passive immunity except in cases of Hib.

| Box 1 |
| Conditions and circumstances that require a customized approach to immunization |

Allergy

Pregnancy

Preterm infancy

Breastfeeding

Immunocompromised state

TST

Severe illness

Cochlear implant

Cerebrospinal fluid leak

Human immunodeficiency virus infection

End-stage renal disease

Chronic heart or lung disease

Chronic liver disease

Diabetes

Asplenia

Complement deficiency

Health care personnel

Men who have sex with men

Data from Hamborsky J, Kroger A, Wolfe S. General recommendations on immunization. In: Hamborsky J, Kroger A, Wolfe S, editors. Epidemiology and prevention of vaccine-preventable diseases. 13th edition. Washington, DC: Public Health Foundation; 2015.

Immunocompromised State

An immunocompromised state can result from congenital immunodeficiency, human immunodeficiency virus (HIV), leukemia, lymphoma, or other generalized malignancy. It can also be caused by chemotherapy agents and chronic use of corticosteroids. A severely immunosuppressed individual should not receive live vaccinations because uncontrolled replication of the vaccine virus could prove overwhelming and even fatal. They may also manifest a diminished response to inactivated vaccines. Consider obtaining antibody titers to confirm immunity.

Tuberculin Skin Testing

The MMR vaccine may reduce the immune response to a tuberculin skin test. The vaccine and test should be administered either at the same time or the TST should be delayed by 4 weeks.

Severe Illness

Severe illnesses have not been found to impair vaccine efficacy or increase the risk of adverse reactions. Despite this, in the presence of severe illness, an adverse vaccine reaction could hinder or complicate diagnosis and treatment of the illness. Therefore, it is acceptable to delay vaccination until the patient has recovered from a severe illness. Mild illness is not an indication for delayed immunizations.

IMMUNIZATION SCHEDULE

It is important for health care providers to know which vaccines are indicated to ensure maximal immunization coverage for each patient. The Advisory Committee for Immunization Practices, under the authority of the CDC, publishes updated immunization schedules on an annual basis, detailing the appropriate age ranges and administration intervals for each scheduled vaccine. These recommendations are found online at www.cdc.gov/.[10] A simplified reference for routine vaccines, grouped by patient age and typical clinic visit intervals, is shown in **Table 2**.[10]

Additional information specific to each vaccine is listed alphabetically in the following sections. Detailed approaches to immunizations in the setting of specific chronic diseases, immunocompromised states, and other risk factors is beyond the scope of this article, as is the recommended catch-up schedule for each specific vaccine. Refer to the current CDC immunization schedule for more information.

VACCINATIONS
Diphtheria, Tetanus, and Acellular Pertussis

Overview
Diphtheria, tetanus, and pertussis are bacterial causes of infection that were relatively common before the advent of their associated vaccines. Diphtheria most commonly affects the pharynx and tonsils, and can be complicated by myocarditis and neuritis with a fatality rate of 5% to 10%. Pertussis initially presents as a common cold but is later associated with paroxysmal coughing spells and an inspiratory whoop. It is most commonly complicated by secondary bacterial pneumonia; seizures and encephalopathy can also occur. Tetanus occurs via contaminated wound transmission. Fatal in 11% of persons affected, it is characterized by a descending pattern of trismus, stiff neck, dysphagia, and rigidity of abdominal muscles.

Currently, the incidences of tetanus and diphtheria are at historic lows with vaccine efficacy virtually 100% for tetanus and 97% for diphtheria. Vaccine efficacy for pertussis is 98% for children 1 year following a 5-dose series but wanes over time, warranting periodic boosters.[11,12]

Recommendations
- Diphtheria, tetanus, acellular pertussis (DTaP) is a 4-dose series administered at 2, 4, 6, and 15 to 18 months of age, followed by booster dose at age 4 to 6 years.
- Tetanus, diphtheria, pertussis (Tdap) is a single dose administered at age 11 to 12 years. All adults, at any age, who have not yet received a dose, should receive a single dose.
- Tetanus, diphtheria (Td) booster is a single dose administered every 10 years after Tdap. It may be recommended for wound management if more than 5 years has passed from the last dose.

Special considerations
- DTaP is contraindicated in patients who develop encephalopathy within 7 days of a prior DTaP dose.
- Tdap should be given during each pregnancy at 27 to 36 weeks' gestation.

Haemophilus influenza Type B

Overview
Haemophilus influenza Type B (Hib) is a bacterial cause of several invasive and potentially severe diseases primarily affecting children younger than 5 years of age. These

Table 2
Immunization schedule by age group

Age	Recommended Routine Vaccinations
Neonate	Hepatitis B (Hep B)
2 mo	Hep B RV1 (2-dose series) or RV5 (3-dose series) Diphtheria, tetanus, acellular pertussis (DTaP) Hib Pneumococcal conjugate vaccine (PCV13) Inactivated poliovirus (IPV)
4 mo	RV1 or RV5 DTaP Hib PCV13 IPV
6 mo	Hep B RV5 (for 3-dose series only) DTaP Hib (for 4-dose series only) PCV13 IPV Inactivated influenza vaccine (IIV)
12 mo	Hib PCV13 MMR Varicella (VAR) Hep A IIV (annual)
15–18 mo	DTaP Hep A (>6 mo after first dose)
4–6 y	DTaP IPV MMR VAR IIV (annual)
11–12 y	Meningococcal (MenACWY) Tetanus, diphtheria, acellular pertussis (Tdap) HPV (2-dose or 3-dose series) IIV (annual)
16 y	MenACWY
≥19 y	IIV (annual) Tdap (1 dose, then tetanus, diphtheria [Td] booster every 10 y) MMR VAR (2 doses separated by >4 wk) HPV (if no prior, not indicated after age 26 y)
≥50 y	IIV (annual) Recombinant zoster vaccine (RZV) (2 doses separated by >8 wk)
≥65 y	IIV (annual) If no prior RZV, 2-dose RZV (preferred) or 1-dose zoster vaccine live (ZVL) PCV13 PPSV23 (1 y following PCV13)

Data from Centers for Disease Control and Prevention. Immunization schedules. Available at: https://www.cdc.gov/vaccines/schedules/index.html. Accessed April 18, 2018.

include meningitis, epiglottitis, pneumonia, arthritis, and cellulitis. It is estimated that the incidence of Hib infections has declined by more than 99% since the prevaccine era, most significantly with the advent of the conjugate Hib vaccine. Clinical efficacy of the vaccine is determined to be 95% to 100%.[13]

Recommendations

- A 3-dose series should be administered at 2, 4, and 12 months of age.
- A 4-dose series also includes a dose at 6 months of age.
- The preferred dose interval is 8 weeks; the minimal interval is 4 weeks.
- The minimal age is 6 weeks.

Special considerations

- Additional doses may be necessary in immunocompromised or asplenic patients.

Hepatitis A

Overview

Hepatitis A (Hep A) infection is often manifest by an abrupt onset of fever, malaise, anorexia, abdominal pain, and jaundice. It can result in both hepatic and extrahepatic complication. The most severe is fulminant hepatitis, which has a mortality rate of 80%. Since vaccine implementation in 1996, Hep A rates have declined 93.7% overall.[14]

Recommendations

- A 2-dose series should be administered starting at 12 months of age, separated by 6 to 18 months, and preferably completed before child's second birthday.
- Adults with risk factors may receive either the 2-dose series of Hep A (doses separated by 6 months) or the 3-dose series of combined Hep A and hepatitis B (Hep B) (doses at 0, 1, and 6 months).

Special considerations

- Hep A risk factors include
  - Travel to endemic countries
  - Men who have sex with men
  - Illicit drug use (injection or noninjection)
  - Laboratory work with Hep A virus
  - Clotting factor disorders
  - Chronic liver disease
  - Contact with an international adoptee
  - Recent exposure to Hep A virus (for adults age 40 and younger).

Hepatitis B

Overview

The Hepatitis B (Hep B) virus is a common cause of viral hepatitis. Transmission occurs via parenteral or mucosal exposure to blood or serous fluids. In the United States, this occurs most commonly in the perinatal period or through sexual contact. This infection can result in fulminant hepatitis (with a 63%–93% fatality rate) or, should it become chronic, will substantially increase a patient's risk for cirrhosis and/or hepatocellular carcinoma and their related mortality. From 1990 to 2004, Hep B incidence in the United States dropped by 75% with the most significant decline (94%) noted in children and adolescents, coinciding with an increase in vaccination coverage.[15,16]

Recommendations

- A 3-dose series should be administered at birth, 1 to 2 months, and 6 months of age.
- A fourth dose is permitted if switching to combination vaccine containing Hep B after birth dose.
- Interval for first and second dose is at least 4 weeks.
- The interval for second and third dose is at least 8 weeks.
- Ensure at least 16 weeks between first and third doses in adults.
- Ensure at least 24 weeks between first and final dose in small children.

Special considerations

- Use only monovalent Hep B in infants less than 6 weeks of age.
- For infants born to a Hep B surface antigen-positive mother, Hep B immune globulin treatment is also indicated.

Human Papillomavirus

Overview

Human Papillomavirus (HPV), the most common sexually transmitted infection in the United States, is closely linked to the incidence of cervical cancer. Other clinical manifestations include anogenital warts, recurrent respiratory papillomatosis, cervical cancer precursors, and other cancers (anal, oropharyngeal, penile, vaginal, and vulvar.) From the more than 140 types of HPV that have been identified, types 16 and 18 have been associated with 66% of cervical cancers. Five additional types (HPV 31, 33, 45, 52, and 58) account for another 15% of all cervical cancers. Types 6 and 11 are associated with 90% of anogenital warts. The HPV vaccine is 99% immunogenic 1 month after completing either dosing series.[17]

Recommendations

- A 2-dose series is recommended for all male and female adolescents at 11 to 12 years of age, spaced by 6 months.
- A 3-dose series is recommended for all adolescents who initiate vaccine at 15 years of age or older, dosed at 0, 1 to 2, and 6 months.

Special considerations

- The 9-valent HPV vaccine covers types 6, 11, 16, 18, 31, 33, 45, 52, and 58, and is currently the only HPV vaccine distributed in the United States.
- This vaccine has no proven therapeutic effect on existing HPV infection, genital warts, or cervical lesions.
- A series may be started as early as age 9 years in cases of sexual abuse or assault, or in immunocompromised persons.
- It is not recommended during pregnancy.

Influenza

Overview

Influenza A and B viruses cause seasonal flu epidemics. Transmission occurs via respiratory droplets and is extremely contagious. Flu symptoms can start 1 to 4 days after acquiring infection. Symptoms are similar to a viral upper respiratory infection but also manifests systemically; particularly with fever, major fatigue, headaches and body aches. The CDC estimates that influenza has resulted in between 9.2 million and 35.6 million illnesses, between 140,000 and 710,000 hospitalizations, and has ranged from a low of 12,000 deaths to a high of 56,000 deaths since 2010.[18,19]

Recommendations

- All persons aged 6 months and older should be vaccinated annually.
- Children aged 6 months through 8 years, during their first season of influenza vaccination, should receive 2 doses, separated by 4 or more weeks.
- There are 3 preparations to choose from:
  - Inactivated influenza vaccines are most commonly given; a high dose administration is recommended for adults 65 years or older.
  - Intranasal live attenuated influenza vaccines were not used during the 2017 to 2018 influenza season due to inefficacy against influenza A (H1N1)pdm09 viruses in the preceding years.
  - Recombinant influenza vaccines are indicated in persons aged 18 years or older with severe egg allergies.[20]

Special considerations

- A typical flu season extends from October to May in the United States.
- It takes 2 weeks for the body's immune system to develop immunity against influenza A and B.
- Persons at high risk for complications related to influenza infections (**Box 2**)[21] should be strongly encouraged to receive the vaccine.
- Studies have shown no true contraindication to receiving a flu vaccine for those with egg allergies. Persons with prior severe allergic reactions (not including anaphylaxis) after exposure to eggs should receive the flu vaccine in a supervised health care setting.[22]

Box 2
Priority people for flu vaccination

Children age 6 months through 4 years

Adults age 50 years or older

People with chronic diseases

Immunocompromised patients

Women who are or will be pregnant during the influenza season, including up to 2 weeks following delivery

Residents of nursing homes and chronic-care facilities

American Indians or Alaska Natives

Morbid obesity (body mass index >40)

Health care personnel

Household contacts and caregivers of high-risk patients

Data from Centers for Disease Control and Prevention. Vaccination: who should do it, who should not and who should take precautions. Available at: https://www.cdc.gov/flu/protect/whoshouldvax.htm. Accessed April 24, 2018.

Measles, Mumps, Rubella, and Varicella

Overview

Measles, mumps, rubella, and varicella are viral diseases with potentially serious sequelae that were very common before vaccinations. They are each highly contagious and primarily transmitted by respiratory droplets. Severe complications have been noted with these infections, including deafness, pneumonia, encephalitis, meningitis, pancreatitis, and birth defects. Estimates from the World Health Organization suggest 17.1 million lives have been saved since 2000 due to MMR vaccination. Two doses of MMR vaccine are 97% effective against measles and 88% effective against mumps. One dose of MMR vaccine is 93% effective against measles, 78% effective against mumps, and 97% effective against rubella. Two doses of the varicella vaccine are 90% effective in producing immunity.[9,23–25]

Recommendations

- A 2-dose series should be administered at 12 months and 4 to 6 years of age.
- A varicella vaccine is given on the same schedule and may be administered separately or in combination with MMR.

Special considerations

- The MMR vaccine contains live attenuated viruses and should not be given to immunocompromised patients or to women known to be or attempting to become pregnant.
- Because of increased risk for febrile seizures, the combined MMRV should be avoided in children younger than 47 months of age.

Meningococcal Disease

Overview

Neisseria meningitides bacterial infection, characterized by fever, headache, and stiff neck, can potentially lead to severe meningitis with 10% to 15% fatality rates and/or meningococcemia with 40% fatality rates. Almost all invasive disease occurrences are caused by 5 of the 13 meningococcal serogroups: A, B, C, W, and Y. Since the late 1990s, the incidence of meningococcal disease has declined across all vaccine-contained serogroups (A, B, C, W, Y) and across all age groups.[26]

Recommendations

- Meningococcal quadrivalent ACWY conjugate vaccines (MenACWY)
  - A 2-dose series is routinely administered at ages 11 to 12 and 16 years.
  - It may be administered earlier in children at an increased risk for meningococcal disease.
  - Adult dosing may be considered in the presence of risk factors (see later discussion), as well as for military recruits and first-year college students living in residential housing who did not receive the MenACWY at age 16 years.
  - Booster doses are indicated every 5 years if risks remain.
- Meningococcal serogroup B (MenB) recombinant vaccines
  - These should be administered only to persons at increased risk for meningococcal disease, aged 10 years and older.
  - Two or 3 doses may be administered depending on vaccine used.[27]

Special considerations

- Meningococcal risk factors include
  - Anatomic or functional asplenia
  - HIV infection
  - Sickle cell disease
  - Persistent complement component deficiency
  - Eculizumab use
  - Laboratory work with *Neisseria meningitides*
  - Travel to endemic countries
  - Exposure during disease outbreak.

Pneumococcal Disease

Overview

Streptococcus pneumoniae is a major bacterial cause of pneumonia, bacteremia, and meningitis. There were 92 serotypes identified as of 2011, 10 of which account for approximately 62% of invasive pneumococcal disease, such as bacteremia and meningitis, worldwide. It results in an estimated 400,000 hospitalizations per year for pneumonia in the United States, with an associated 5% to 7% fatality rate. Fatality rates increase to more than 20% in cases of invasive disease, which occur mostly in young children, the elderly, and the immunocompromised.

Two vaccines are currently available in the United States. The first, pneumococcal conjugate vaccine, PCV13, covers 13 serotypes of pneumococcus, accounting for 61% of invasive disease among children less than 5 years of age. It is 90% effective against invasive disease in children. For adults older than age 65 years, it is 45% effective against pneumonia and 75% effective against invasive disease. The second, PPSV23, covers 23 serotypes, accounting for 60% to 76% of bacteremic pneumococcal disease. It is ineffective in children younger than age 2 years. For adults older than age 65 years, it is 60% to 70% effective against invasive disease but no significant impact has been confirmed in the prevention of pneumonia.[28]

Recommendations

- For infants, PCV13 should be administered at 2, 4, 6, and 12 months of age.
- For adults 65 years and older, a single dose of PCV13 is recommended, followed by a single dose of PPSV23 at least 1 year later.
- Consider earlier and additional doses in patients with risk factors for pneumococcal infection, as well as booster doses for persons with continuing risk.

Special considerations

- PCV13 should be dosed before PPSV23 when possible.
- Pneumococcal risk factors include
  - Chronic disease
  - Anatomic or functional asplenia
  - Immunocompromised state
  - Alcoholism
  - Cerebrospinal fluid leaks
  - Cochlear implants
  - Cigarette smoking.

Poliovirus

Overview
Poliovirus infections enter the body orally and, following an incubation period of 1 to 3 weeks, can spread to the motor nerve fibers. Between 1% to 5% infected persons will develop nonparalytic aseptic meningitis symptoms. Less than 1% will develop paralysis, which, depending on the severity and if the brainstem is involved, can be fatal. Since the introduction of the polio vaccine, endemic cases of paralytic polio have dropped from a high of 20,000 annually in the 1950s to none occurring since 1979.[29]

Recommendations
- Four-dose series should be administered at 2, 4, and 6 months, and at 4 to 6 years of age.

Special considerations
- Routine vaccination of adults greater than 18 years is not recommended unless travel to polio-endemic countries is anticipated.
- Oral polio vaccine is no longer approved for use in the United States due to risk for vaccine-associated paralytic polio.

Rotavirus

Overview
Rotavirus is a significant cause of viral gastroenteritis, especially in children aged 6 months to 2 years of age. It is transmitted via the fecal-oral route and is characterized by vomiting, nonbloody diarrhea, and fever. In severe cases dehydration, seizures, and death can occur. Since the vaccine was reintroduced in 2006, rotavirus-related hospitalization and emergency department visits among children younger than 5 years has reduced by 67% across the globe.[30,31]

Recommendations
- Attenuated human RV1, in a 2-dose series, should be administered at 2 and 4 months of age.
- Pentavalent human-bovine rotavirus reassortant vaccine (RV5), in 3-dose series, should be administered at 2, 4, and 6 months of age.

Special considerations
- In premature infants, administer after 6 weeks of age.
- Prior rotavirus gastroenteritis infection does not confer complete immunity. Proceed with vaccination series.
- It is contraindicated in children with SCID.

Varicella-Zoster Virus

Overview
Varicella-zoster virus, the cause of chicken pox, is highly contagious and primarily transmitted by respiratory droplets. Reactivation of the dormant varicella virus within dorsal root ganglia results in herpes zoster (shingles). An estimated 1 million episodes of zoster occur in the United States annually with an overall lifetime individual risk estimated at 32%. This condition can be complicated by the development of persistent postherpetic neuralgia or other sequelae, depending on the location and organs infected. The varicella vaccine reduces the incidence of zoster 69.8% in persons 50

to 59 years old and by 51% in persons 60 to 80 years old, as well as significantly reduces the risk of postherpetic neuralgia.[9]

Recommendations

- For adults age greater than 50 years, recombinant zoster vaccine (RZV) should be administered in 2 doses, 2 to 6 months apart.
- For adults age older than 60 years without prior zoster vaccination, either 2 doses of RZV (preferred) or a single dose of zoster vaccine live (ZVL) may be administered.

Special considerations

- ZVL is contraindicated in pregnant or severely immunocompromised patients.

SUMMARY

Vaccination is among the most effective preventative health measures in modern times. It has positively affected the incidence and prevalence of a myriad of diseases, as well as improved both their morbidity and mortality. It is essential that health care providers understand the value of this intervention, promote comprehensive immunization coverage within their community, and recognize the underlying principles that guide decisions regarding vaccination. Factors important to consider before immunization administration include the type of vaccination, its recommended timing and intervals, and the presence of contraindications, precautions, or other special considerations.[32,33]

REFERENCES

1. Andre FE, Booy R, Bock HL, et al. Vaccination greatly reduces disease, disability, death and inequity worldwide. Bull World Health Organ 2008;86(2):81–160.
2. Hamborsky J, Kroger A, Wolfe S, editors. Epidemiology and prevention of vaccine-preventable diseases. 13th edition. Washington, DC: Public Health Foundation; 2015.
3. Vaccine types. US Department of Health & Human Services Web site. Available at: https://www.vaccines.gov/basics/types/index.html. Accessed June 13, 2018.
4. Ehreth J. The global value of vaccination. Vaccine 2003;21(7–8):596–600.
5. Vaccine-preventable disease morbidity in the United States. Centers for Disease Control and Prevention Web site. 2018. Available at: https://www.cdc.gov/ncird/surveillance/materials-resources.html. Accessed June 13, 2018.
6. Hamborsky J, Kroger A, Wolfe S. General recommendations on immunization. In: Hamborsky J, Kroger A, Wolfe S, editors. Epidemiology and prevention of vaccine-preventable diseases. 13th edition. Washington, DC: Public Health Foundation; 2015. p. 09–27.
7. Klein NP, Fireman B, Yih WK, et al. Measles-mumps-rubella-varicella combination vaccine and the risk of febrile seizures. J Pediatr 2010;126(1):e1–8.
8. Vaccine adverse event reporting system. US Dept of Health and Human Services. Available at: https://vaers.hhs.gov/. Accessed April 25, 2018.
9. Hamborsky J, Kroger A, Wolfe S. Varicella. In: Hamborsky J, Kroger A, Wolfe S, editors. Epidemiology and prevention of vaccine-preventable diseases. 13th edition. Washington, DC: Public Health Foundation; 2015. p. 327.

10. Immunization schedules. Centers for disease control and prevention web site. 2018. Available at: https://www.cdc.gov/vaccines/schedules/index.html. Accessed April 18, 2018.
11. About diphtheria, tetanus, and pertussis vaccines. Centers for Disease Control and Prevention Web site. 2016. Available at: https://www.cdc.gov/vaccines/vpd/dtap-tdap-td/hcp/about-vaccine.html. Accessed April 23, 2018.
12. US Dept of Health and Human Services. Updated recommendations for use of tetanus toxoid, reduced diphtheria toxoid, and acellular pertussis (Tdap) vaccine in adults aged 65 years and older–Advisory Committee on Immunization Practices (ACIP), 2012. Morb Mortal Wkly Rep 2012;61(25):468–70.
13. Hamborsky J, Kroger A, Wolfe S. *Haemophilus influenza* type b. In: Hamborsky J, Kroger A, Wolfe S, editors. Epidemiology and prevention of vaccine-preventable diseases. 13th edition. Washington, DC: Public Health Foundation; 2015. p. 119–29.
14. Hamborsky J, Kroger A, Wolfe S. Hepatitis A. In: Hamborsky J, Kroger A, Wolfe S, editors. Epidemiology and prevention of vaccine-preventable diseases. 13th edition. Washington, DC: Public Health Foundation; 2015. p. 136–46.
15. Hamborsky J, Kroger A, Wolfe S. Hepatitis B. In: Hamborsky J, Kroger A, Wolfe S, editors. Epidemiology and prevention of vaccine-preventable diseases. 13thedition. Washington, DC: Public Health Foundation; 2015. p. 149–65.
16. Schillie S, Vellozzi C, Reingold A, et al. Prevention of Hepatitis B virus infection in the United States: recommendations of the advisory committee on immunization practices. Morb Mortal Wkly Rep 2018;67(No. RR-1):1–31.
17. Meites E, Kempe A, Markowitz LE. Use of a 2-dose schedule for human papillomavirus vaccination — updated recommendations of the advisory committee on immunization practices. Morb Mortal Wkly Rep 2016;65:1405–8.
18. Disease burden of influenza. Centers for Disease Control and Prevention Web site. 2018. Available at: https://www.cdc.gov/flu/about/disease/burden.htm. Accessed April 24, 2018.
19. Manzoli L, Schioppa F, Boccia A, et al. The efficacy of the influenza vaccine for healthy children; a meta-analysis evaluating potential sources of variation in efficacy estimates including study quality. Pediatr Infect Dis J 2007;26:97–106.
20. Grohskopf LA, Sokolow LZ, Olsen SJ, et al. Prevention and control of influenza with vaccines: recommendations of the advisory committee on immunization practices, United States, 2015-16 influenza season. MMWR Morb Mortal Wkly Rep 2015;64(30):818–25.
21. Vaccination: who should do it, who should not and who should take precautions. Centers for Disease Control and Prevention Web site. 2017. Available at: https://www.cdc.gov/flu/protect/whoshouldvax.htm. Accessed April 24, 2018.
22. Flu vaccine and people with egg allergies. Centers for Disease Control and Prevention Web site. 2017. Available at: https://www.cdc.gov/flu/protect/vaccine/egg-allergies.htm. Accessed April 24, 2018.
23. Hamborsky J, Kroger A, Wolfe S. Measles. In: Hamborsky J, Kroger A, Wolfe S, editors. Epidemiology and prevention of vaccine-preventable diseases. 13th edition. Washington, DC: Public Health Foundation; 2015. p. 209–25.
24. Hamborsky J, Kroger A, Wolfe S. Mumps. In: Hamborsky J, Kroger A, Wolfe S, editors. Epidemiology and prevention of vaccine-preventable diseases. 13th edition. Washington, DC: Public Health Foundation; 2015. p. 247–56.
25. Hamborsky J, Kroger A, Wolfe S. Rubella. In: Hamborsky J, Kroger A, Wolfe S, editors. Epidemiology and prevention of vaccine-preventable diseases. 13th edition. Washington, DC: Public Health Foundation; 2015. p. 325–38.

26. Hamborsky J, Kroger A, Wolfe S. Meningococcal disease. In: Hamborsky J, Kroger A, Wolfe S, editors. Epidemiology and prevention of vaccine-preventable diseases. 13th edition. Washington, DC: Public Health Foundation; 2015. p. 231–41.

27. Patton ME, Stephens D, Moore K, et al. Updated recommendations for use of MenB-FHbp Serogroup B meningococcal vaccine — advisory committee on immunization practices, 2016. MMWR Morb Mortal Wkly Rep 2017;66:509–13.

28. Hamborsky J, Kroger A, Wolfe S. Pneumococcal disease. In: Hamborsky J, Kroger A, Wolfe S, editors. Epidemiology and prevention of vaccine-preventable diseases. 13th edition. Washington, DC: Public Health Foundation; 2015. p. 279–92.

29. Hamborsky J, Kroger A, Wolfe S. Poliomyelitis. In: Hamborsky J, Kroger A, Wolfe S, editors. Epidemiology and prevention of vaccine-preventable diseases. 13th edition. Washington, DC: Public Health Foundation; 2015. p. 297–306.

30. Burnett E, Jonesteller CL, Tate JE, et al. Global impact of rotavirus vaccination on childhood hospitalizations and mortality from diarrhea. J Infect Dis 2017;215(11): 1666–72.

31. Hamborsky J, Kroger A, Wolfe S. Rotavirus. In: Hamborsky J, Kroger A, Wolfe S, editors. Epidemiology and prevention of vaccine-preventable diseases. 13th edition. Washington, DC: Public Health Foundation; 2015. p. 311–21.

32. Robinson CL, Romero JR, Kempe A, et al. Advisory committee on immunization practices recommended immunization schedule for children and adolescents aged 18 years or younger — United States, 2018. MMWR Morb Mortal Wkly Rep 2018;67:156–7.

33. Kim DK, Riley LE, Hunter P. Advisory committee on immunization practices recommended immunization schedule for adults aged 19 years or older — United States, 2018. MMWR Morb Mortal Wkly Rep 2018;67:158–60.

Screening

Pediatric Screening
Development, Anemia, and Lead

Sarah K. Wood, MD, FAAP*, Randi Sperling, DO, FAAP, FACOP

KEYWORDS

- Pediatric screening • Child development • Developmental disorders
- Iron deficiency • Lead poisoning

KEY POINTS

- Primary care providers play a critical role in pediatric preventive health care and must be aware of important screening recommendations to ensure comprehensive health supervision as children grow and develop.
- Routine pediatric screening varies by patient age and risk factors.
- Developmental surveillance and screening help to identify delays at an earlier age.
- Iron deficiency remains a significant public health problem requiring screening for at-risk pediatric patients.
- Approaches to the care of patients with lead poisoning include prevention, screening of those at high risk, environmental changes, and treatment in select patients.

INTRODUCTION

Primary care providers play a critical role in pediatric preventive health care and must be aware of important screening recommendations to ensure comprehensive health supervision as children grow and develop. Many valuable resources have been developed to assist providers in identifying developmental, nutritional, and psychosocial risk factors for disease. The American Academy of Pediatrics (AAP) and Bright Futures provide summary consensus recommendations in a Pediatric Periodicity Schedule that make available the timing of screenings, procedures, and appropriate anticipatory guidance recommended for each age-based visit during childhood.[1] This article addresses prevention and screening for 3 major childhood health problems, namely, developmental concerns, iron deficiency anemia, and lead poisoning.

Disclosure Statement: The authors have nothing to disclose.
Division of Pediatrics, Department of Integrated Medical Sciences, Charles E. Schmidt College of Medicine, Florida Atlantic University, 777 Glades Road, Building 71, Boca Raton, FL 33431, USA
* Corresponding author.
E-mail address: SWood31@health.fau.edu

Prim Care Clin Office Pract 46 (2019) 69–84
https://doi.org/10.1016/j.pop.2018.10.008
0095-4543/19/© 2018 Elsevier Inc. All rights reserved.

primarycare.theclinics.com

DEVELOPMENT

Pediatric primary care providers are uniquely positioned to provide critical developmental surveillance throughout childhood at periodic well-child visits. Serving as the medical home for children necessitates the incorporation of standardized developmental surveillance and screening to identify developmental concerns. The timely identification of developmental problems is essential because it can lead to the diagnosis of underlying medical, behavioral, psychosocial, and developmental disorders that will benefit from early identification and treatment. Developmental surveillance should be part of every routine checkup, and when any concerns are raised, appropriate follow-up screening tests should be recommended. Routine developmental screening tests should be administered at the 9-, 18-, and 24- or 30-month visits. Besides playing an important role in the early diagnosis of developmental delays, primary care providers should coordinate care by optimizing referrals, providing follow-up visits, and working collaboratively with early intervention and other professional specialty care providers.

Epidemiology

The prevalence of developmental or behavioral disorders in the United States is high, with approximately 13% of children having a developmental disability. Data from the Centers for Disease Control and Prevention and the Health Resources and Services Administration shows that in 2006 to 2008, 1 in 6 children in the United States had a developmental disorder. Research also reveals that the prevalence of developmental disabilities increased 17.1% from 1997 to 2008, yet only 21% of parents report that their child actually received developmental screening by a health care provider.[2] This finding highlights the critical need for primary care providers to be educated on the screening, diagnosis, treatment, and coordination of care for families impacted by these disorders.

Developmental Surveillance

Development encompasses the physical, cognitive, and socioemotional growth that occurs throughout the transition from infancy to adulthood. Developmental components include behavioral, psychological, and physical concerns, and incorporate the broad domains of gross motor skills, fine motor skills, and cognitive, language, and communication skills, as well as social and emotional skills. A comprehensive, evidence-based, developmental surveillance and screening process must be thoughtfully put in place in all primary care practices to identify children at risk. The AAP recommends that all children undergo developmental surveillance at every well-child checkup throughout infancy, childhood, and adolescence, as well as targeted developmental–behavioral screening at ages 9, 18, and either 24 or 30 months.[3] Surveillance includes taking a complete medical and family history, asking parents whether they have any particular concerns about their child, assessing for developmental risk factors, assessing for protective factors, measuring developmental milestones, and performing a complete physical examination to evaluate for any underlying medical issues (**Box 1**). In taking a full medical and family history at every checkup, it is important that primary care providers include a routine series of open-ended questions on development (**Box 2**).

It must be underscored that any parental concerns should be followed up on with an evidence-based developmental screening tool, but the absence of any concerns does not preclude the presence of a developmental issue. It is the responsibility of the health care professional to continue to evaluate all aspects of the child, including

---

Box 1
Comprehensive developmental surveillance for children at well-child checkups

- A full history including reviewing the child's complete past medical, social, developmental, and family history, and identifying developmental risk factors.
- Asking the parents about the child's most recent developmental accomplishments and whether they have any concerns about their child's developmental progression.
- Observing the child and completing a full age-appropriate physical examination.
- Providing anticipatory guidance that highlights what developmental milestones the family should be expecting next.
- Using appropriate developmental screening tests as recommended by the American Academy of Pediatrics.
- Offering educational resources to families to support healthy development.
- Documenting and maintaining a comprehensive medical record that outlines the development of the child.

---

ongoing developmental surveillance and screening, and to provide reassurance only after a thorough assessment has been completed.

Assessing developmental risk factors
Successful child development is the result of many synergistic factors that work in coordination to allow for appropriate social, emotional, cognitive, and motor progression throughout infancy and childhood. Poverty, malnutrition, an unstable home environment, or lack of intellectual, emotional, or educational support can profoundly impact developmental outcomes.[4] A previsit survey or history taking related to the topics listed in **Box 3** may help identify children at risk owing to psychosocial and medical risk factors. Protective factors can also be elicited particularly focusing on resilience and positive parenting styles.

Monitoring developmental milestones
Primary care providers are strongly encouraged to develop a system of milestone checklists within their offices to support documentation of developmental milestones at each patient's well-child checkup. Reviewing these checklists with parents at the visit can encourage open discussion and education.

Complete physical examination
The physical examination is part of every health supervision visit. The primary care provider should be sure to complete an age-appropriate, comprehensive

---

Box 2
Questions to ask during a developmental history

- What new things has your child begun to do since his/her last visit? (Provide some age-appropriate examples, such as crawling, walking, pointing.)
- Are you comfortable with how your child is developing?
- Are you comfortable with how your child is behaving?
- Do you have any questions about your child's development? Or any concerns?
- Do you have any worries about your child's vision, hearing, behavior, or ability to learn?

Box 3
Developmental risk factors

Medical risk factors

- Prematurity
- Small for gestational age or other prenatal or perinatal complication
- Anemia
- Lead poisoning
- Congenital heart disease
- Neurologic disease
- Hypothyroidism
- Down syndrome
- Hypothyroidism
- Other acute and chronic illnesses

Psychosocial risk factors

- Low level of education
- Poverty (particularly with housing/food instability)
- History of mental health problems (particularly depression or anxiety)
- Unemployed parent
- Single parent household
- Limited literacy
- Concerning parenting characteristics

---

physical examination on each child with attention to aspects of the physical examination that relate to the development of behavioral or developmental disorders.

Laboratory Evaluation

Laboratory screening should be performed as recommended for health supervision including evaluation for iron deficiency and lead poisoning. For infants, newborn metabolic screening testing should be reviewed. Additional laboratory tests or imaging tests may be indicated based on the clinical findings from the history and physical examination (eg, thyroid function testing, genetic testing, metabolic testing, electroencephalography, MRI).

Developmental Screening

The AAP recommends that all children undergo general developmental screening at their well-child checkups at 9 months, 18 months, and either 24 or 30 months. This screening involves the administration of a brief standardized survey that helps to identify children at risk of a developmental disorder. Most screening tools can be completed by parents and then scored by a member of the health care team, often a nonphysician. There are a variety of developmental screening tools available for practitioners to select from including but not limited to the Parents' Evaluations of Developmental Status, the Ages and Stages Questionnaire-3, and the Parents' Evaluations of Developmental Status—Developmental Milestones. The responsible physician should review and interpret the results of the screening tool. If a child has risk factors for developmental concerns, for example, prematurity, then additional screening tests may be necessary. **Box 4** outlines what should be included during developmental screening checkups as recommended by the AAP and Bright Futures.

Autism-Specific Screening

The AAP also recommends autism-specific screening at ages 18 and 24 months using one of many validated tools. The Modified Checklist for Autism in Toddlers, Revised with Follow-Up, is a commonly used tool that helps to identify children at risk for autism spectrum disorders in children ages 16 and 30 months. The Modified Checklist for Autism in Toddlers, Revised with Follow-Up is available through the official Modified Checklist for Autism in Toddlers website.[5] The first part of the 2-step tool is a 20-question survey for parents that takes about 5 minutes to complete. The second part is a follow-up questionnaire administered by the health care provider. It asks the same questions as part 1, over 5 to 10 minutes, but allows the practitioner to further investigate at-risk responses noted. High-risk behaviors and early symptoms concerning for autism include parental concerns about their child's social skills, language skills, and/or behavior (such as frequent temper tantrums, resistance to change, delayed

---

Box 4
Recommended visits for developmental screening in children

9 months

- Administer a general developmental tool/survey selected and reviewed by the health care provider.
- Inquire what motor milestones the child has reached.
- Inquire what communication and language milestones the child has reached.
- Inquire about risk factors for autism, for example, eye contact, receptive language, pointing.
- Inquire whether the parents have any concerns about the child's vision, hearing, or behavior.
- If child is at risk or seems to have a developmental delay refer immediately for evaluation.
- Provide anticipatory guidance to families and review upcoming expected milestones.

18 months

- Administer a general developmental tool/survey selected and reviewed by the health care provider.
- Administer a developmental tool specifically to assess the child's risk for autism.
- Inquire what motor, communication, and language milestones the child has reached.
- If child is at risk or seems to have a developmental delay refer immediately for evaluation.
- Provide anticipatory guidance to families and review upcoming expected milestones.

24/30 months

- Administer a general developmental tool/survey selected and reviewed by the health care provider.
- Administer a developmental tool specifically to assess the child's risk for autism.
- Inquire what motor, communication, and language milestones the child has reached.
- If child is at risk or seems to have a developmental delay refer immediately for evaluation.
- Provide anticipatory guidance to families and review upcoming expected milestones.

or regressed language skills). Specifics such as no babbling by 9 months, no pointing or indicating gestures by 12 months, no single words by 16 months, no pretend or symbolic play by 18 months, and no 2-word phrases by 2 years. There are many additional tests besides the Modified Checklist for Autism in Toddlers, Revised with Follow-Up, available to screen for autism, including but not limited to the Early Screening of Autistic Traits, Screening Tool for Autism in Toddlers and Young Children, Childhood Autism Spectrum Test, and Autism Spectrum Screening Questionnaire.

Patients identified to be at high risk for a developmental disorder should be rapidly referred to a local early intervention program. These programs are extremely valuable when a child is referred early so that patients and their families may receive developmental therapies, coordination of care, and financial support, as well as family support and education. A specific developmental disorder does not need to be diagnosed before an early intervention referral being made. The AAP policy statement on "Care Coordination in the Medical Home: Integrating Health and Related Systems of Care for Children with Special Health Care Needs" highlights the critical importance of an effective partnership with the early intervention team to facilitate successful coordination of care for children with developmental delays. They suggest that parents' complete development screening tools/surveys in the waiting room or online before the appointment, and then a clinical staff member review the screening tool results. If a child is less than 3 years old and at risk then they should be referred immediately to early intervention services. If a child is greater than 3 years old and at risk, then they should be immediately referred to special education services. If the developmental screening tool is negative and the child does not seem to be at risk or have delays, then they should be rescreened at the next appropriate well-child visit. This process allows developmental screening to be effectively and efficiently integrated into a pediatric primary care office, and referrals to be made in a timely manner.

Development Summary

All pediatric health care professionals must embrace the responsibility of serving as the primary care medical home for children and providing children and families with appropriate screening for developmental problems. Every well-child checkup should include developmental surveillance, and standardized developmental screening tools should be used when surveillance identifies a child who is high risk, and for all children at their 9-, 18-, and 30-month visits. Patients identified with developmental concerns should be referred to early development services and effective coordination of care for families should be prioritized to ensure optimal outcomes.

IRON DEFICIENCY ANEMIA
Clinical Description of Disease

Anemia is a decrease in the number of red blood cells (RBCs) and hemoglobin (Hgb) concentration in the blood (**Box 5**). RBCs contain iron, which is needed to produce Hgb, and are vital because they provide oxygen to the body. When there is not enough iron, Hgb production is decreased, which then affects the number of RBCs, causing anemia. The causes of anemia are typically categorized into disorders that result in an increased rate of RBC destruction, a decreased rate of RBC production, or RBC loss secondary to acute or chronic bleeding.

Iron deficiency anemia is a global health problem and a common medical condition seen in everyday pediatric clinical practice. Iron deficiency occurs when there is not enough iron, or the iron stores in the body are depleted. Iron, the most abundant trace

---

Box 5
Pathophysiology of anemia

Inadequate production of red blood cells

  Vitamin deficiencies

  Iron deficiency anemia

  Chronic disease

  Bone marrow disease

  Aplastic anemia

  Transient erythropenia of childhood

Destruction of red blood cells

  Sickle cell anemia

  Hemolytic anemia

  Mechanical injury

  Hemolytic –uremic syndrome

  Hemangioma

  Enzyme defects

Glucose-6-phosphate dehydrogenase

  Blood loss

  Acute bleeding

  Chronic bleeding

---

element in the body, is needed to produce Hgb and is necessary for oxygen transport. Iron is stored in the liver, spleen, and bone marrow, and the transport of iron in the body is mediated by 3 proteins. These proteins are:

- Transferrin (iron transport protein)
- Transferrin receptor 1 (TFR1)
- Ferritin (iron storage protein)

Iron is transported from the duodenum into the mucosal cells of the stomach in the ferrous state, where it is then converted into the ferric state it either combines with apoferritin to form ferritin or crosses into the plasma. In the plasma, iron is bound to transferrin, then delivered to the bone marrow, where it binds to receptors on the RBC. It then releases iron into the ferrous state. Iron absorption occurs mostly in the duodenum and the upper jejunum and is influenced by various factors. In the diet, iron can be found in both animal and plant sources. The best sources of iron are usually those acquired from animal products because it contains heme iron, which is found in the RBC.

Signs and symptoms of iron deficiency anemia are listed in **Box 6**. Other syndromes associated with iron deficiency anemia include restless leg syndrome as well as breath holding spells. Cognitive defects and behavioral abnormalities have been linked to iron deficiency anemia. However, it has been difficult to establish a causal relationship between iron deficiency anemia and cognitive deficits because of the many confounding variables and the difficulty in designing and executing the large, randomized, controlled trials necessary to distinguish small potential differences. In a study by

---

Box 6
Signs and symptoms of iron deficiency anemia

- Fatigue
- Poor appetite
- Pale skin, conjunctiva, mucous membranes, and nailbeds
- Slowed growth and development
- Tachypnea
- Unusual cravings for ice, dirt, paint (pica)
- Brittle nails
- Cheilosis

McCann and Ames,[6] which reviewed the evidence of a causal relationship between iron deficiency/iron deficiency anemia and deficits in cognitive and behavioral function, there was at least some support for causality with iron deficiency anemia. However, because the specificity for both cause and effect have not been established unequivocally, it is hard to determine whether there is an existence of a causal relationship between iron deficiency anemia and cognitive and behavioral performance.

Epidemiology

The incidence of iron deficiency anemia in children has decreased significantly over the past several decades, primarily owing to iron fortification of infant formulas and cereals. Iron-fortified formula was recommended by the AAP in 1969 and adopted into the WIC program in the 1970s. However, iron deficiency anemia remains a common cause of anemia and nutritional deficiency among children. The prevalence of iron deficiency anemia in children ages 1 to 3 years in the United States ranges from 8% to 14%. Some studies have shown that there is an increased incidence of iron deficiency anemia in African Americans (1.6%), Mexican Americans (0.9%), children living below the poverty line (2.2%), and WIC recipients (3.1%).

Other factors that might increase a child's risk for iron deficiency anemia include:

- Prematurity,
- Low birth weight,
- Use of non–iron-fortified formula,
- Introduction of cow's milk before 1 year of age,
- Exclusive breastfeeding without supplementation,
- Exposure to increased levels of lead,
- Chronic health problems,
- Restricted diets, and
- Greater than 24 oz cow's milk per day in the diet.

Full-term infants have iron stores that last for approximately 4 to 6 months, with the stores being depleted by 6 to 9 months, and iron deficiency becoming apparent by 9 to 12 months of age. The iron in cow's milk has lower bioavailability than human breast milk (5%–10% vs 50% absorption) and Milk can potentially interfere with the absorption of iron present in other foods. Cow's milk has the ability to damage the intestinal mucosa, leading to blood loss. Children less than 24 months of age are at greatest risk for iron deficiency anemia because of rapid growth and the change from breastmilk or iron-fortified formula to cow's milk and a regular diet that might not supply all of the needed nutritional benefits. Adolescent girls are also at high risk because of blood loss through menstruation, rapid growth, and poor diets.

Screening Guidelines

The aim of screening for iron deficiency anemia in young children is to identify and treat anemia before it leads to poor health outcomes. Parameters of the complete blood count that are necessary to examine are the Hgb, the mean corpuscular volume (MCV), and the red cell distribution width (RDW). The Hgb and the mean corpuscular volume would be low in iron deficiency anemia, whereas the red cell distribution width would be increased.

The AAP guidelines indicate that screening should occur in all children between 9 months and 1 year of age (**Boxes 7** and **8**). The Hgb and hematocrit are inexpensive laboratory tests that are rapid and easy to perform; however, the sensitivity and specificity vary significantly depending on the population and the reference standards used. Although capillary sampling might be easier than venous blood sampling, the results are less reliable, because obtaining blood from a fingerstick might cause hemolysis and contaminate the blood with tissue fluids. Abnormal capillary samples should be confirmed with venous blood testing. Currently, there is no single measurement that will characterize the iron status of a child. To identify iron deficiency or iron deficiency anemia, the Hgb concentration should be combined with other measurements of iron status.

Some tests that may be added to the Hgb concentration include serum ferritin, reticulocyte Hgb content (CHr), and TFR1. The serum ferritin is a sensitive parameter for measurement of iron stores in healthy subjects. A value of 10 μg/L has been suggested as a minimum value. However, because serum ferritin is an acute phase reactant, concentrations may be increased in the presence of chronic inflammation, infection, malignancy, or liver disease. Combining the serum ferritin with a C-reactive protein level might be a reliable testing measure if the C-reactive protein is not elevated owing to inflammation. The CHr and TFR1 levels are not affected by inflammation, malignancy, or anemia of chronic disease, and might be preferable. The CHr assay measures the iron available to cells recently released from the bone marrow. A low CHr concentration is a strong predictor of iron deficiency in children and might be useful for diagnosis when the assay becomes more available. TFR1 is a measure of iron status, detecting iron deficiency at the cellular level. TFR1 is found on cell membranes and facilitates the transfer of iron into the cells. When there is an inadequate supply of iron, there is an upregulation of TFR1 and enables the cells to compete for iron. An increase in TFR1 concentration is seen in patients with iron

---

Box 7
Iron deficiency anemia screening

- Test Hgb concentration at 9 months to 1 year of age
- Confirm abnormal capillary samples with venous blood samples
- Consider combining hemoglobin testing with serum ferritin and C-reactive protein level if appropriate
- Other tests to consider
  - Reticulocyte hemoglobin content (currently being investigated, assay not readily available)
  - Transferrin receptor 1 (currently being investigated, assay not readily available)

Box 8	
Laboratory results consistent with a diagnosis of iron deficiency anemia	
Hemoglobin	↓
Hematocrit	↓
Mean corpuscular volume	↓
Red cell distribution width	↑
Peripheral smear	Microcytosis, hypochromia, decreased red blood cells
Serum iron studies	Iron and ferritin decreased
Total iron binding capacity	↑
Transferrin receptor 1	↑
Hemoglobin electrophoresis	Normal
Response to iron supplementation	Increase in hemoglobin

deficiency anemia, although it does not increase if serum iron stores are completely depleted. The TFR1 assay is not widely available and the standards for infants and children have not been established.

To establish a diagnosis of iron deficiency anemia, one can measure a serum ferritin and C-reactive protein level or a CHr level. A Hgb concentration of less than 11 g/dL would need to be present as well. Another approach that has been used clinically in children with mild anemia (Hgb 10–11 g/dL) is to monitor the response to iron supplementation, especially if, by history, the diet is iron deficient. An increase of 1 g/dL after 1 month of therapeutic supplementation is usually diagnostic. This supplementation of iron requires patient compliance in taking the medication. Supplementation should not be used to diagnose patients who have problems with iron absorption.

Prevention Recommendations

Iron can be obtained through natural food sources such as meat, poultry, and legumes. Nonheme iron vegetarian diets are less well-absorbed and might have higher iron requirements. The recommended dietary allowance of iron for infants ages 7 to 12 months is 11 mg/d and in 1- to 3-year-old children, 7 mg/d. The preterm infant (<37 weeks of gestation) who is breastfed should receive a supplement of elemental iron at 2 mg/kg/d starting at 1 month of age and continuing until 1 year of age. Preterm infants who are fed a standard preterm infant formula or a standard term infant formula will receive approximately 1.8 to 2.2 mg/kg/d of iron, assuming a formula intake of 150 mL/kg/d. Despite the use of iron-containing formula, 14% of preterm infants develop iron deficiency anemia between 4 and 8 months of age. Some formula-fed infants might need additional iron supplementation, although currently there is not enough evidence to make a general recommendation. Term breast fed infants usually have sufficient iron stores until 4 to 6 months of age. The World Health Organization recommends exclusive breastfeeding for 6 months, whereas the AAP recommends exclusive breastfeeding for a minimum of 4 months, preferably 6 months.

Dietary prevention

- Iron supplementation with foods rich in iron-such as pureed meats, beans, and iron-fortified cereals should be initiated between 4 and 6 months of age.
- In toddlers, once they have switched to cow's milk, it is important to limit intake to 20 to 24 ounces/d.
- Vitamin C helps with the absorption of iron, so foods rich in this vitamin such as citrus fruit, cantaloupes, tomatoes, and strawberries should be included in the diets of toddlers.

Outcomes

Iron deficiency in infancy might lead to subsequent poor neurocognitive development; however, screening and early treatment have not consistently improved neurocognitive outcomes. It is possible that the prevention of neurodevelopmental consequences of iron deficiency anemia may require the prevention of iron deficiency, rather than the detection and treatment of existing iron deficiency. Another possibility is that the prevention of neurodevelopmental consequences may require screening and early treatment of multiple nutritional deficiencies, rather than iron deficiency alone.

Complications

The potential harm associated with screening for iron deficiency anemia might be the risk of false positive results, as well as the cost involved. The potential harms of treatment for iron deficiency anemia would include the possibility of GI side effects, as well as the risk of unintentional overdose.

Iron Deficiency Anemia Summary

Iron deficiency anemia remains a significant public health concern requiring screening of pediatric patients. More accurate testing measures are currently being evaluated. Dietary interventions during rapid periods of growth, as well as supplementation for at-risk patients might help in the prevention of iron deficiency anemia.

LEAD
Clinical Manifestations of Disease

Lead, a natural element found in the environment, has been known to have harmful effects on children. Children are exposed to lead from different sources such as soil, dust, air, food, and water. The clinical presentation of lead poisoning can vary, depending on the age of the patient, as well as the amount and duration of exposure. Lead is absorbed from the gastrointestinal tract more efficiently in younger children, so they are at higher risk of symptoms owing to lead poisoning. When the neurologic system is affected, children can experience:

- Behavioral changes,
- Hyperactivity,
- Lower IQ scores,
- Loss of language and developmental milestones,
- Severe toxicity can lead to seizures and encephalopathy, and
- Other clinical manifestations include nausea, vomiting, abdominal pain, pica, constipation, anorexia, as well as renal manifestations.

Anemia can develop with lead poisoning, secondary to impaired synthesis of heme. Symptoms of lead poisoning are typically nonspecific and may vary owing to differences in individual susceptibility and environmental exposures.

Epidemiology

In the United States, according to the Centers for Disease Control and Prevention, an estimated 310,000 children younger than 5 years of age have elevated lead levels greater than 5 μg/dL in the blood.[7] With the elimination of lead from paint and gasoline over the past few decades, lead levels in most children have decreased significantly. Common sources of lead exposure are listed in **Box 9**. Race and ethnicity have been linked to higher rates of lead poisoning, with non-Hispanic blacks and Mexican

---

Box 9
Common sources of lead exposure

- Lead paint
- Dust
- Water
- Ceramics
- Folk medications

Americans at much higher risk than non-Hispanic whites. Children from households below the federal poverty level are also more likely to have elevated lead levels. Other children at risk include those who live in homes in a zip code with a high percentage of reported lead poisoning (**Box 10**).

Diagnostic Screening

Although substantial environmental improvements have been made to decrease exposure to lead, prevention, as well as screening of high-risk children is highly recommended. It is important to obtain an environmental exposure history to see if the exposure to lead can be eliminated. The overall sensitivity of the questionnaires designed to identify lead poisoning in children is about 60% to 70%. Screening is recommended to begin no later than 1 year of age, repeated as needed, and then again performed at 2 years of age. This is an important age to screen because of the infant's increased mobility, as well as the hand to mouth activity at this stage of development.

Obtaining a blood lead level is necessary for diagnosis. Venous blood levels are preferred over capillary samples, because environmental lead contamination of the skin can lead to false-positive results. If a capillary lead level is elevated, it needs confirmation with a venous sample.

- High-risk children, including immigrants, children living below the poverty level, refugees, and international adoptees, should be screened.
- All children enrolled in Medicaid are required to receive blood lead screening tests at ages 12 and 24 months (**Box 11**).
- In addition, any child between the ages of 24 and 72 months, with no record of a previous blood lead screening test must receive one.

In 2012, Centers for Medicare and Medicaid Services expanded its lead screening policy to allow states to request approval from Centers for Medicare and Medicaid Services for a targeted screening program.[8] The current Bright Futures/AAP

Box 10
Risk factors for increased lead levels

- Living in or visiting a house with peeling paint
- Lower socioeconomic level
- High-risk zip codes
- Living in or visiting homes built before 1978, especially if in process of remodeling
- Siblings/playmates with increased lead levels

Box 11
Lead screening guidelines

- Check lead levels for all children receiving WIC/Medicaid at 1 and 2 years of age.
- Check children between the ages of 2 and 6 years of age who were not previously screened.
- Administer risk questionnaires at 6 months, 9 months, 1 year, 1.5 years, 2 years, and 3 to 6 years of age.
- If positive risk assessment, check lead levels.

Periodicity Schedule recommends a lead risk assessment at the 6-month, 9-month, 12-month, 18-month, 24-month, and 3- to 6-year well-child visits. The current recommendation is to perform a risk assessment and to obtain a blood lead level only if the risk assessment comes back positive. According to the AAP and Centers for Disease Control and Prevention, universal screening tests of blood lead levels are not recommended except for high prevalence areas and increased risk factors. A reference level of 5 μg/dL has now been established to identify children with blood lead levels that are much higher average. The new level is based on the US population of children ages 1 to 5 years who are in the highest 2.5% of children tested for increased lead levels. Any child found to have a blood venous lead level of greater than 5 μg/dL requires follow-up blood testing. Elevated blood lead levels are to be reported to the state's department of health.

Lead Poisoning Prevention Recommendations

Clinicians play an important role in the prevention of childhood lead exposure. Screening questionnaires, as well as educating patients and families to minimize exposure to lead, is important in preventive health care. Specific nutritional anticipatory guidance that may decrease the incidence of lead toxicity, such as encouraging an adequate intake of calcium, vitamin C, and iron, should be discussed at well-child visits. Clinicians should also question about the condition of the home environment and ask about any planned renovations.

Outcomes

Blood lead concentrations have been decreasing in children in the United States owing to environmental improvements, and the incidence of fatal lead encephalopathy has essentially disappeared. Although there are guidelines for managing children with increased lead levels, it is important to continue to focus on preventative measures and education.

Complications

Falsely elevated lead level results may be caused by contaminants of the tube or poor laboratory methodology. Capillary screening might underestimate the true blood lead level if the finger is squeezed to obtain the sample. Lead does not remain in the blood for long periods of time, so blood lead levels do not exclude the possibility of substantial bone lead levels.

Lead Summary

Lead poisoning remains one of the most common diseases of environmental origin among US children. Secondary prevention of lead poisoning through screening and treatment will remain necessary as long as children continue to be exposed to lead.

Early detection of elevated lead levels is important to ensure lead abatement occurs, thereby minimizing morbidity from lead poisoning.

SUMMARY

Preventive health services and screening can help detect risk factors, diseases, and disorders earlier, therefore benefiting the overall health of the child. Pediatric primary care providers must stay current with screening guidelines as well as be aware of available tools and resources to enhance the care of their patients. The AAP and Bright Futures Pediatric Periodicity Schedule are extremely valuable and comprehensive resources that should be used as a guide for practitioners because they address developmental, behavioral, and nutritional concerns in their practices.

REFERENCES

1. Hagan JF, Shaw JS, Duncan PM, editors. Bright Futures: Guidelines for Health Supervision of Infants, Children, and Adolescents. 4th ed. Elk Grove Village, IL: American Academy of Pediatrics; 2017. Available at: https://brightfutures.aap. org/materials and tools/guidelines-and pocketguide. Accessed April 25, 2018.
2. Centers for Disease Control and Prevention/Child Development/Developmental Disabilities. Available at: https://www.cdc.gov/ncbddd/childdevelopment/index/ html. Accessed April 25, 2018.
3. Bright Futures. 4th edition. Itasca (IL): AAP; 2017.
4. Ali SS. A brief review of risk-factors for growth and developmental delay among preschool children in developing countries. Adv Biomed Res 2013;2:91.
5. M-CHAT. What is the M-CHAT test? Available at: https://mchat.org. Accessed April 25, 2018.
6. McCann JC, Ames BN. An overview of evidence for a causal relation between iron deficiency during development and deficits in cognitive or behavioral function. Am J Clin Nutr 2007;85(4):931–45.
7. Centers for Disease Control and Prevention (CDC). Lead. Available at: https:// www.cdc.gov/lead. Accessed April 25, 2018.
8. Centers for Medicare & Medicaid Services. Lead screening. Available at: www. medicaid.gov.lead. Accessed April 25, 2018.

FURTHER READINGS

GENERAL SCREENING

Bright Futures guidelines. 4th edition. American Academy of Pediatrics; 2017. Available at: https://brightfutures.aap.org/materials and tools/guidelines-and pocketguide. Accessed April 25, 2018.

WEBSITES

American Academy of Pediatrics (AAP). Available at: http://www2.aap.org/sections/ dbpeds/practice-screening.asp.
Birth to Five: Watch Me Thrive. Available at: www.hhs.gov/watchmethrive.
Bright Futures. Available at: www.brightfutures.org.
Centers for Disease Control and Prevention (CDC). Use of selected clinical preventive services to improve health of infants, children, and adolescents – United States, 1999-2011. Available at: www.cdc.gov/mmwr/pdf/other/su6302.pdf.

Centers for Disease Control and Prevention (CDC). CDC's "Learn the Signs. Act Early." program. Available at: www.cdc.gov/actearly.

Centers for Medicare & Medicaid Services. Lead screening. Available at: www.medicaid.gov.

Child and Adolescent Health Measurement Initiative. Available at: www.childhealthdata.org.

Health Resources & Services Administration (HRSA). Early Periodic Screening, Diagnosis, and Treatment Program (EPSDT) and Title V. Available at: http://mchb.hrsa.gov/epsdt/index.html.

M-CHAT revised with follow-up. Available at: https://m-chat.org/.

National Survey of Children's Health. Available at: https://www.cdc.gov/nchs/slaits/nsch.htm.

New York State Department of Health. Sources of lead. Available at: www.health.ny.gov/environmental/lead.

DEVELOPMENT

Accardo PJ, Whitman BY, Behr SK, et al. Dictionary of developmental disabilities terminology. 2nd edition. Baltimore (MD): Paul H. Brookes Publishing Co; 2003.

American Academy of Pediatrics Council on Children with Disabilities. Care coordination in the medical home: integrating health and related systems of care for children with special health care needs. Pediatrics 2005;116:1238–44.

Centers for Disease Control and Prevention (CDC). Child development. Developmental disabilities. Available at: https://www.cdc.gov/ncbddd/childdevelopment/index.html; https://www.cdc.gov/ncbddd/developmentaldisabilities/features/birthdefects-dd-keyfindings.html. Accessed November 12, 2017.

Council on Children with Disabilities, Section on Developmental Behavioral Pediatrics, Bright Futures Steering Committee, Medical Home Initiatives for Children with Special Needs Project Advisory Committee. Identifying infants and young children with developmental disorders in the medical home: an algorithm for developmental surveillance and screening. Pediatrics 2006;118(1):405–20.

Dworkin PH. British and American recommendations for developmental monitoring: the role of surveillance. Pediatrics 1989;84:1000–10.

Glascoe FP, Dworkin PH. The role of parents in the detection of developmental and behavioral problems. Pediatrics 1995;95:829–36.

Glascoe FP. The value of parents' concerns to detect and address developmental and behavioural problems. J Paediatr Child Health 1999;35:1–8.

Pulsifer MB, Hoon AH, Palmer FB, et al. Maternal estimates of developmental age in preschool children. J Pediatr 1994;125:S18–24.

ANEMIA

Baker RD, Greer FR, Committee on Nutrition American Academy of Pediatrics. Diagnosis and prevention of iron deficiency and iron-deficiency anemia in infants and young children (0-3 years of age). Pediatrics 2010;126(5):1040–50.

Biondich PG, Downs SM, Carroll AE, et al. Shortcomings in infant iron deficiency screening methods. Pediatrics 2006;117(2):290–4.

Brotanek JM, Gosz J, Weitzman M, et al. Iron deficiency in early childhood in the US; risk factors and racial ethnic disparities. Pediatrics 2007;120(3):374–81.

Brugnara C, Adamson J, Auerbach M, et al. Iron deficiency- what are future trends in diagnosis and therapeutics. Clin Chem 2013;59(5):740–5.

Helfand M, Freeman M, Nygren P, et al. Screening for iron deficiency anemia in childhood and pregnancy: update of 1996 USPSTF review and evidence synthesis 40 (prepared by the Oregon Evidence Based Practice Center under contract No. 290-02-0024. Rockville (MD): Agency for Healthcare Research and Quality; 2006.

Iannotti LL, Tielsch JM, Black MM, et al. Iron supplementation in early childhood: health benefits and risks. Am J Clin Nutr 2006;4(6):1261–76.

Irwin J, Kirchner J. Anemia in children. Am Fam Physician 2001;64(8):1379–87.

Lozoff B, Jimenez E, Hagan J, et al. Poorer behavioral and developmental outcome more than 10 years after treatment for iron deficiency in infancy. Pediatrics 2000;105(4):e51.

Martins S, Logan S, Gilbert R. Iron therapy for improving psychomotor development and cognitive function in children under the age of 3 with iron deficiency. Cochrane Database Syst Rev 2001;(2):CD001444.

Mocan H, Yildiran A, Orhan F, et al. Breath holding spells in 91 children and response to treatment with iron. Arch Dis Child 1999;81(3):261–2.

Powers J, Buchanan G. Iron deficiency anemia in toddlers to teens: how to manage when prevention fails. Contemp Pediatr 2014;31(5):12–7.

Short M, Domajalski J. Iron deficiency anemia: evaluation and management. Am Fam Physician 2013;87(2):98–104.

Ullrich C, Wu A, Armsby C, et al. Screening healthy infants for iron deficiency using reticulocyte hemoglobin content. JAMA 2005;294:924–30.

US Preventive Series Task Force. Screening for iron deficiency anemia, including iron supplementations for children and pregnant women: recommendation statement. Am Fam Physician 2006;74(3):461–4.

LEAD

American Academy of Pediatrics Committee on Environmental Health. Screening for elevated blood lead levels. Pediatrics 1998;101:1072–8.

American Academy of Pediatrics Committee on Environmental Health. Lead exposure in children: prevention, detection, and management. Pediatrics 2005;116(4):1036–46.

Bennett K, Lowry J, Newman N. Lead poisoning: what's new about an old problem? Contemp Pediatr 2015.

Centers for Disease Control and Prevention (CDC).. Blood lead levels–United States 1999-2002. MMWR Morb Mortal Wkly Rep 2005;54(20):513–6.

Centers for Disease Control and Prevention (CDC). CDC Childhood lead poisoning prevention program. National surveillance data 1997-20D11. Atlanta (GA): US Department of Health, Centers for Disease Control and Prevention; 2014.

Centers for Disease Control and Prevention (CDC). Lead. Available at: https://www.cdc.gov/lead/. Accessed January 5, 2001.

Chadridan L, Cataldo R. Lead poisoning: basics and new developments. Pediatr Rev 2010;31:399.

Lowry JA, Paulson JA, American Academy of Pediatrics Committee on Environmental Health. Lead exposure in children: prevention, detection and management. Pediatrics 2005;116(4):1036–46.

Markowitz M. Lead poisoning. Pediatr Rev 2000;21(10):327–35.

Theppeang K, Glass TA, Bandeen-Roche K, et al. Gender and race/ethnicity differences in lead dose biomarkers. Am J Public Health 2008;98(7):1248–55.

Warniment C, Tsang K, Galazka SS. Lead poisoning in children. Am Fam Physician 2010;81(6):751–7.

Geriatrics Screening and Assessment

Mandi Sehgal, MD*, Elizabeth Hidlebaugh, MD, Matthew G. Checketts, DO, Bernardo Reyes, MD

KEYWORDS

- Geriatric • Screening • Assessment

KEY POINTS

- Geriatric screening and assessment is critical for maximizing the health, function, safety, and quality of life of older patients.
- Reversible and treatable conditions are often underdiagnosed and undertreated in geriatric patients.
- Assessing function and quality of life is crucial in older adults.
- Knowledge of a patient's goals, values, and preferences combined with an understanding of their social history, social supports and living circumstances are essential to providing person-centered care.

INTRODUCTION

Worldwide, older adults are living with chronic, complex illness that affects all aspects of their lives. Clinicians must understand how to provide compassionate, high-quality care to this population. This article provides a framework to using standard geriatric screening questions and assessment tools as a complement to the standard history and physical examination.

RECOMMENDATIONS FOR GERIATRIC SCREENING AND ASSESSMENT

The purpose of geriatric screening and assessment is to identify concerns in the following domains: social, functional, geriatric syndromes, and cognition and affect[1] (**Table 1**) with the intent to capture and formulate them into a person-centered context with a plan to deliver safe and effective care.

Disclosure Statement: The authors have nothing to disclose.
Department of Integrated Medical Science, Florida Atlantic University, Charles E. Schmidt College of Medicine, 777 Glades Road, BC 71, Boca Raton, FL 33431, USA
* Corresponding author.
E-mail address: sehgalm@health.fau.edu

Table 1
Recommendations for geriatric screening and assessment

Geriatric Assessment Domains		Screening Questions	Further Geriatric Assessment for Positive Responses to Screening
SOCIAL	Social Support	• Do you live alone? • Are you looking for someone to help with your daily activities? • Are you a caregiver for someone?	• Consider referral to a social worker or a local Area Agency on Aging • Lubben Social Network Scale, Revised
	Alcohol Abuse	• Do you drink > 2 drinks / day?	• AUDIT-5
	Elder Neglect/Abuse	• Do you ever feel unsafe where you live? • Has anyone ever threatened or hurt you? • Has anyone been taking your money without your permission?	• Consider referral to a social worker and/or Adult Protective Services • Elder Abuse Suspicion Index
	Advance Directives	• Do you have a power of attorney for health care (DPAHC) or a living will? • Have you thought about the type of care you would want if you become seriously ill?	• Advance care planning discussion • Execute a document, e.g. a DPAHC or Physician Orders for Life-Sustaining Treatment (POLST) or similar form
FUNCTIONAL	Functional Status	• Do you need assistance with shopping or finances? • Do you need assistance with bathing or taking a shower?	• Instrumental ADL Assessment • Basic ADL Assessment
	Driving	• Do you still drive? If yes: • While driving, have you had an accident in the past 6 months? • Are any family members concerned about your driving?	• Vision testing • Consider a formal driving evaluation
	Vision	• Do you have trouble seeing, reading, or watching TV? (with glasses, if used)	• Vision testing • Consider referral for eye exam
	Hearing	• Do you have difficulty hearing conversation in a quiet room? (with aid if used) • Whisper Test	• Check for cerumen in ear canals and remove if impacted • Hearing Handicap Inventory • Consider Audiology referral
GERIATRIC SYNDROMES	Polypharmacy	• Do you take 5 or more routine medications (excluding vitamins and other supplements)? • Do you understand the reason for each of your medications?	• Perform medication reconciliation, match medications to diagnoses • Consider reducing doses, stopping drugs, adherence aides, and/or consultation with a pharmacist
	Fall Risk	• Have you fallen in the past year? • Are you afraid of falling? • Do you have trouble climbing stairs or rising from a chair?	• "Get Up and Go" test • Consider full Fall Assessment • Consider Physical Therapy Evaluation • Consider Home Safety Assessment
	Incontinence	• Do you have any trouble with your bladder? • Do you lose urine or stool when you do not want to? • Do you ever wear pads or adult diapers?	• Consider 3-IQ Questionnaire (women) or AUASS symptom inventory (men) • Consider continence evaluation
	Weight Loss	• Have you lost 10 or more pounds over the last 6 months without intending to do so? • Weight <100 pounds?	• Assess for risk factors for malnutrition • Consider evaluation by a dietician/nutritionist
	Sleep Disturbance	• Do you often feel sleepy during the day? • Do you have difficulty falling asleep at night? • Do you snore loudly?	• Consider a sleep scale (e.g. Pittsburgh Sleep Index) • Consider referral for sleep evaluation
	Pain	• Are you experiencing pain or discomfort?	• Pain Assessment using a standard scale
COGNITION AND AFFECT	Depression	• Do you often feel sad or depressed? • Have you lost pleasure in doing things over the past few months?	• Perform PHQ – 9 or Geriatric Depression Scale • Screening for suicide risk • Consider psychology or psychiatry evaluation
	Cognitive Impairment	• Do you or any family or friends think you have a problem with your memory? • Confusion Assessment Method (CAM) to screen for delirium • Mini Cog (3-item recall, clock draw)	• If Mini Cog failed, test with a standard tool (e.g. MoCA, SLUMS, MMSE) • Consider neuropsychological testing, if diagnosis is unclear

Adapted from Kane RL, Ouslander JG, Resnick B, et al. Evaluating the geriatric patient. In: Edmonson KG, Yoo C, editors. Essentials of clinical geriatrics. 8th edition. New York: McGraw-Hill; 2018. p. 52–3; with permission.

Social Domain

Social support

A person's social wellbeing can influence overall health. It is important to differentiate between the need for support with daily living tasks, which are often provided by family or caregivers, and emotional support, which is often provided by close friends.

There is an association between increased social support and reduced risk of physical disease and mental illness,[2] and, for those with chronic illnesses, increased survival and quality of life.[3] Clinicians should not only encourage social interaction but should also screen for its absence. Screening questions can include "Do you live alone?," "Are you looking for someone to help with your daily activities?," and "Are you a caregiver for someone?"[1]

What constitutes appropriate social support is challenging for clinicians to determine because what may be adequate for 1 patient may not be enough for another. The Lubben Social Network Scale, Revised,[4] measures self-reported social engagement, including family and friends, and correlates with mortality, all cause hospitalization, health behaviors, depressive symptoms, and overall physical health.

Alcohol abuse
Defining alcohol abuse is challenging in older adults. Alcohol abuse is common among older adults, yet frequently goes unrecognized.[5] A standard screening question is "Do you drink 2 or more drinks per day?"[1] Additionally, another valuable source of information is a history from family or caregivers.

In older adults, small amounts of alcohol can lead to symptoms of intoxication, resulting in adverse outcomes, including major injuries. Symptoms of alcohol abuse can be nonspecific (eg, falls, cognitive impairment), and may lead to a diagnosis that fails to include alcohol use in the differential. Often the diagnosis of alcohol abuse focuses on issues such as not fulfilling major obligations, recurrent legal problems and social isolation, which may lead to underdiagnosis in older adults who may have limited social interactions or are retired.[6] Instruments used to screen for problem drinking and potential alcohol abuse include the most widely known and studied, CAGE questionnaire[7] and the Alcohol Use Disorders Identification Test (AUDIT)-5.[8]

Elder abuse
Defined as intentional or neglectful actions by a caregiver or a trusted individual that could result in harm to an older adult, elder abuse occurs most often in domestic settings. Spouses and male children are the most common perpetrators of elder abuse.[9] Clinicians should be aware of the possibility of abusive or neglectful behavior and screen for it during each visit.

Screening questions for elder abuse include "Do you ever feel unsafe where you live?," "Has anyone threatened or hurt you?," and "Has anyone taken your money without your permission?"[1]

Clinicians should look for physical examination findings such as burns, weight loss, poor hygiene, and pressure injuries. Those suffering from abuse may present with nonspecific signs and symptoms that could be confused with the effect of chronic illness; for example, weight loss in patients with advanced dementia or injuries among patients with a history of previous falls. Special care needs to be taken when screening patients for abuse because they may be afraid to discuss abusive behaviors due to fear of repercussions from family or caregiver and/or being removed from their current environment. A patient who sits quietly in the office, avoids eye contact, and hesitates to answer questions in front of family members should be interviewed in private. The Elder Abuse Suspicion Index[10] is a standard tool used to augment a history regarding potential abuse. Clinicians should be aware of the specific requirements to report elder abuse in the state in which they practice.

Advance directives
Advance directives allow patients to maintain autonomy during permanent or temporary incapacity. The most common types of advance directives are the living will and the durable power of attorney for health care.

Initiating the discussion of advance directives can be challenging. Screening questions include "Do you have a power of attorney for health care or a living will?" and "Have you thought about the type of care you would want if you became seriously ill?"[1]

A discussion about advance directives should take into account the patient's goals and values, which are often inextricably linked to their cultural background. They should not be limited to establishing wishes regarding the use of cardiopulmonary resuscitation if needed (code status). Discussion should include preferences regarding treatment options and, if the patient wishes, should include family or caregivers, with the goal of better understanding the patient's preferences for their care.

Patients who have advance directives are less likely to receive unnecessary and unwanted care at the end of life. Patients are more likely to discuss advance directives with clinicians whom they have an established relationship; many think it is the responsibility of the clinician to start the conversation.[11] The most effective interventions associated with successful documentation of advance directives involve serial discussions (preferably face-to-face).[12] The use of educational materials also may facilitate the conversation but their effectiveness as a sole intervention is limited.[13]

In the United States, there are ongoing efforts to create consistency of process in the discussion and definitions of planning for end-of-life care that focuses on patients' values and priorities. The Physician Orders for Life-Sustaining Treatment (POLST) form[14] is an example. POLST aims to (1) enhance advance care planning conversations between patients, health care professionals, and families and caregivers and (2) standardize documentation of shared decision-making between a patient and his or her health care providers regarding the patient's treatment preferences.

Discussing advance directives is a dynamic process that evolves with the patient's medical conditions, living situation, and beliefs. Clinicians should be aware of existing advance directives with the purpose of honoring them when there are changes in health status, such as a new diagnosis of a terminal illness or worsening of a chronic condition.

Functional Domain

Functional status

Assessment of activities of daily living (ADL) and instrumental ADL (IADL) are critical in assessing an older adult's functional status (**Table 2**). ADL are self-care activities necessary for daily functioning. IADL are more complex than ADL and, although not necessary for daily functioning, they are critical to allow for independent living. Impairments in ADL or IADL have been associated with postoperative complications, predict functional status decline and mortality,[15] and incur higher hospital costs.[16]

Table 2
Activities of daily living and instrumental activities of daily living

ADL	IADL
Walking	Housekeeping
Transferring: getting in or out of bed or chair	Shopping
	Meal preparation
Bathing	Managing finances
Dressing	Using the telephone
Toileting	Doing laundry
Eating	Using transportation
Continence	Medication management

Screening questions used to identify difficulty with ADL or IADL include "Do you need assistance with shopping or finances?" and "Do you need assistance with bathing or taking a shower?"[1] Shopping and managing finances are 2 higher level IADL that are often impaired first, before others. Similarly, bathing and showering are 2 of the more complex ADL that are likely to be impaired before others. These questions and their subsequent follow-up assessments can be used with patients throughout the health care continuum from the hospital to home. Both the patient and family or caregiver should be asked these questions because the answers often differ.[17]

IADL should be assessed after hospitalization or acute illness, office visits, or with reported changes in physical or cognitive function. One of the most widely used and longstanding IADL assessments is the Lawton IADL Scale.[18] Each IADL is scored based on functional ability (from independently able to perform to unable to perform). It is important to keep in mind gender, age, and cultural and socioeconomic factors that may influence responses to certain questions.[17] For example, certain demographics of older adult men were not often involved in housework; therefore, they may answer that they need assistance with housework.

The most widely used and recognized ADL scale is the index of ADL developed by Katz and colleagues[19] and Katz.[20] It assesses each ADL as they were over the 2 weeks preceding the evaluation and assesses them on a scale from being independent, to needing assistance, to being dependent. The setting in which the patient is being assessed may influence the patient's independence level. For example, hospitalized patients or those in skilled nursing facilities may not be allowed to perform certain ADL for safety reasons.

Driving

Driving allows for a sense of independence and pleasure for many patients. However, older adults have the highest risk of being involved in fatal crashes.[21] Evaluation of an older adults' driving should start with an assessment of (1) the patient's cognition, vision, and hearing; (2) a thorough medication history; and (3) obtaining a driving history from family or caregivers. Reversible causes of poor driving skills should be sought and corrected if possible to avoid unnecessarily taking away a patient's driving privileges. Clinicians should be aware of their state's individual requirements for reporting impaired drivers.[21]

Screening questions about driving include "Do you still drive?" If yes, "While driving, have you had an accident in the past 6 months?" and "Are any family members concerned about your driving?"[1] The best approach to assessing a patient's driving, besides routinely asking patients and caregivers about driving, is a combination of neuropsychological testing and road testing by a trained occupational therapist. A valuable, free resource is the Clinician's Guide to Assessing and Counseling Older Drivers.[22] This guide includes wealth of information on driving assessment and includes patient educational materials.

Vision

Impaired vision is a risk factor for falls, immobility, depression, cognitive decline, and delirium.[23] In the United States, 7% of people aged 65 and older live with vision difficulty or disability.[24] Aging is associated with increased prevalence of eye diseases such as cataracts, age-related macular degeneration, diabetic retinopathy, glaucoma, and presbyopia.[25]

Screening questions to assess for vision impairment include "Do you have trouble seeing, reading, or watching TV (with glasses, if used)?"[1] Medications should be reviewed for those known to cause blurry vision, particularly those with anticholinergic properties. Visual field testing and ophthalmoscopy should also be performed to look for common, correctable eye diseases (eg, cataracts).[26] Further evaluation by an optometrist or ophthalmologist should be considered if the patient is unable to read the letters on or below the 20/40 line on a Snellen eye chart.

Hearing

Hearing impairment is the most common sensory impairment in older adults. Presbycusis affects 30% to 47% of persons older than age 65 years.[26] In the United States, 15% of people aged 65 years and older live with hearing difficulty or disability.[24] As with vision impairment, hearing impairment is a risk factor for delirium and depression and is associated with decreased quality of life, memory, and executive dysfunction. Reversible causes of hearing loss, such as cerumen impaction, should be investigated and treated.[26] The US Preventive Services Task Force (USPSTF) recommendations state that there is insufficient evidence to assess the balance of benefits and harms of hearing screening in asymptomatic adults 50 years and older.[27] If screening is desired, clinicians should ask patients about hearing loss and an affirmative response should prompt further testing. A screening question that can begin the conversation about issues with hearing is, "Do you have difficulty hearing conversation in a quiet room? (With aid if used)."[1]

If a patient or their caregiver is concerned about hearing impairment, after ruling out cerumen impaction, the 10-item Hearing Handicap Inventory for the Elderly (HHIE) should be administered.[28] The HHIE is answered based on how a patient hears without use of a hearing aid and assesses how hearing impairment affects emotional and social adjustment.

A whisper test may also be performed. While covering the nontested ear, the clinician stands at arm's length behind the patient and whispers a combination of 3 numbers and letters and asks the patient to repeat what they heard. This test is performed independently for each ear. The test is positive for decreased hearing if the patient is unable to repeat at least 3 of 6 numbers or letters.[26]

Other in-office testing includes audiometry using a handheld audioscope, which delivers varying tones at variable frequencies. If the patient cannot hear either the 1000 or 2000 Hz frequency in both ears or both the 1000 or 2000 Hz frequencies in 1 ear they should be referred for audiology evaluation.[25]

Geriatric Syndromes

Polypharmacy

As patients develop comorbid conditions, the number of prescribed medications may increase. Polypharmacy is generally defined as 5 or more medications prescribed concomitantly.[1] Medications and patients' understanding of how to take them and what the side effects are should be reviewed at each encounter. Clinicians have the responsibility to be familiar with common medication interactions and adverse effects, and must be vigilant to avoid such adverse events. This information is readily available in many electronic health records and databases.

Screening questions to assess for polypharmacy include "Do you take 5 or more routine medications (excluding vitamins and other supplements)?" and "Do you understand the reason for each of your medications?"[1]

Often, patients will be prescribed a medication and may develop a known side effect of the medication. However, instead of discontinuing this medication, the side effect is treated as a new condition and another medication is prescribed. This is known as the prescribing cascade and often contributes to polypharmacy.[29]

The following questions may help to identify and interrupt the prescribing cascade in practice[29]:

1. Is the new drug being prescribed to treat an adverse effect of a previously prescribed medication?
2. If yes, was the initial drug that had been prescribed a necessity for this patient?
3. What are the pros and cons of continuing the drug therapy that had initiated this prescribing cascade?

Consideration should be given to reduce medication doses to the lowest, most effective doses; stopping medications when appropriate; avoiding potentially adverse drug interactions; and using aides to assist with adherence. There are published guidelines to educate safe prescribing practices, such as the Beer's Criteria[30]; and, there are resources to guide deprescribing. Consultation with a pharmacist can also be beneficial to ensure patients are on the most appropriate medications.

Fall risk

According to the Centers for Disease Control and Prevention (CDC), millions of older adults fall each year but less than half inform their physician. The direct health care costs of falls amount to 31 billion USD annually.[31]

Given that falls are a significant cause of morbidity and mortality, it is critical to screen for fall risk routinely. Screening questions to assess fall risk include "Have you fallen in the past year?," "Are you afraid of falling?," "Do you have trouble climbing the stairs?," and "Do you have trouble getting up from a chair?"[1]

If any of these questions are answered in the affirmative, or in patients presenting with a primary complaint of a fall, a falls assessment, including an evaluation of gait, should be conducted. Stopping Elderly Accidents, Death, and Injury (STEADI)[32] is an online educational resource from the CDC for practicing clinicians and patients.

Urinary incontinence

Urinary incontinence (UI) is the involuntary leakage of urine and is common among older adults, especially women. As many as 50% of American women experience UI over their lifetime.[33] Men may also experience UI, especially those that have undergone prostatectomy. UI affects quality of life, may be embarrassing for the patient, and is often a factor in making the decision to seek nursing home care.[1]

It is important to screen for UI as a routine part of care of older adults because it can affect quality of life and limit function. Screening questions for UI include "Do you have any trouble with your bladder?," "Do you lose urine when you do not want to?," and "Do you ever wear pads or adult diapers?"[1] The 3-Incontinence Questionnaire (3-IQ) for women[34] or the American Urological Association Symptom Score (AUASS) for men[35] can be useful to help assess the type and severity of incontinence.

A history that characterizes specific symptoms that bother the patient and a physical examination should be performed to evaluate UI. Pertinent parts of the physical examination for UI, include abdominal and rectal examinations; genitourinary examination, including a pelvic examination for female patients; and a basic neurologic examination. In addition, a clean-catch urinalysis should be obtained to rule out urinary tract infection as a cause of UI.[1] Most older adults should also have a postvoid residual determination. Specific findings should prompt referral for further evaluation.[1]

Weight loss

Clinically important weight loss is defined as the loss of 10 lb (4.5 kg) or greater than 5% of one's body weight over a period of 6 to 12 months.[36] Unintentional weight loss may be the result of an underlying disease or the first sign of functional decline. It is important to weigh older adult patients at each office visit and to ask appropriate screening questions. Significant weight loss is associated with increased mortality, which can range from 9% to as high as 38% within 1 to 2.5 years in the absence of clinical awareness and attention.[36]

Screening questions for weight loss include "Have you lost weight without trying?"[1] If the patient replies in the affirmative, follow up with, "How much weight have you lost in the past 6 to 12 months?"[1] For established patients, it is important to corroborate their answers based on objective data from the health record and with their family or caregiver. The patient's medication list should be reviewed for medications that can cause anorexia. Oral hygiene, nutrition intake, and access to food should also be assessed. Referral to a dietician should be considered as part of the evaluation of weight loss.

Sleep

Sleep disorders, including insomnia, obstructive sleep apnea, and restless leg syndrome, are among the most common conditions physicians encounter.[37] More than one-half of American adults experience some type of intermittent sleep disturbance.[37]

Screening questions to assess for sleep disturbance include "Do you often feel sleepy during the day?," "Do you have difficulty falling asleep at night?," and "Do you snore loudly?"[1] These questions should be confirmed with the patient's sleep partner when available. Patients who answer affirmatively to these screening questions should have a thorough history and physical examination. Conditions such as pain, gastroesophageal reflux, nocturia, and depression as contributors to sleep disturbance should be considered. The Pittsburgh Sleep Index[38] can help differentiate poor from good sleep quality. Referral for a sleep evaluation should be considered to assist with diagnosing sleep disturbances, especially for those suspected of having sleep apnea because of its associated morbidity.

Pain

Pain is the most common complaint reported by the older adult population to their primary care physicians.[33] The most common cause of persistent pain is musculoskeletal but neuropathic pain and ischemic pain occur frequently, and multiple concurrent causes are often found.[33]

Persistent pain results in restricted activity, depression, sleep disruption, and social isolation, and increases the risk of adverse events due to medication.[33]

Asking, "Are you experiencing pain or discomfort?"[1] is a way to screen for pain. Pain at rest and with specific activity should be identified. Patients with advance dementia may have difficulty articulating their pain, instead manifesting their pain as disruptive behavior.[1] Asking family or caregivers about these behaviors in addition to looking for visual cues (furrowed brows, grimacing, muscle tension, moaning) can be helpful.

Pain should be assessed with a structured history and physical examination, and a standard pain scale should help identify the nature and severity of the pain and help guide diagnosis and treatment. Treatment of pain often requires a multimodal and multidisciplinary approach to care to sustain quality of life and function.

Cognition and Affect Domain

Depression

Depression screening in older adults is important because of this condition's high morbidity. Older adults may not complain of depressive symptoms, and symptoms may be atypical or masked in patients with cognitive impairment or neurologic disorders.[25] The USPSTF and American Academy of Family Physicians recommend screening for depression in the general adult population. The Patient Health

Questionnaire (PHQ)-2[39] is a validated tool and includes 2 questions: "Over the past month, have you often had little interest or pleasure in doing things?" and "Over the past month, have you often been bothered by feeling down, depressed, or hopeless?" The screen is positive with scores of 3 or higher. For each question, score 0 for not at all, 1 for several days, 2 for more than half the days, and 3 for nearly every day.[25] If patients have a positive screen on the PHQ-2, the next step is to use the PHQ-9[40] or the Geriatric Depression Scale[41] and to ask about suicidal thoughts and firearms in the home. The risk of suicide is highest among white men older than 65 years and firearms are the most common method in older adults.[42] A referral to a psychologist or psychiatrist trained in caring for older adults should be considered if the PHQ-9 or Geriatric Depression Scale findings reveal mild to moderate depression. In addition, after discussion of benefits and risks, consideration of the use of an antidepressant may be appropriate in certain patient populations.

Cognitive impairment
In the United States, 9% of people aged 65 years and older live with cognitive difficulty or disability.[24] The USPSTF states that there is insufficient evidence to assess the balance of benefits and harms of cognitive impairment screening in older adults.[43]

A screening question for memory impairment is "Do you or any family or friends think you have a problem with your memory?"[1] If the patient or caregiver endorses memory impairment, after ruling out delirium using the Confusion Assessment Method (CAM),[44] the Mini-Cog[45] should be performed. The CAM is well-validated and includes questions on the acuity of onset, inattention, disorganized thinking, and altered level of consciousness.[44]

The Mini-Cog consists of 3 steps: 3 item recall (max of 3 points) and clock drawing (max of 2 points), and is scored on a 5-point scale.[45] A score of 3 out of 5 is generally considered the cutoff point for cognitive impairment; 4 out of 5 can be used as a cutoff point if greater sensitivity is desired. If patients score a 3 out of 5 on the Mini-Cog, follow-up testing with a standard assessment tool for cognitive impairment such as the Montreal Cognitive Assessment (MoCA),[46] St. Louis University Mental Status Examination (SLUMS),[47] or the Mini Mental Status Exam (MMSE)[48] should be performed. If the diagnosis remains unclear, referral for neuropsychological testing can be helpful. The Gerontological Society of America offers a free online toolkit to assist with evaluating and caring for older adults with cognitive impairment.[49]

To complete the evaluation, a history and physical examination, functional status assessment, computed tomography or MRI of the brain, complete blood count, comprehensive metabolic panel, thyroid-stimulating hormone, vitamin B12, and (if clinically suspected) human immunodeficiency virus and syphilis testing should be performed. Medications should be reviewed for any that may be contributing to cognitive impairment and to identify treatments for anxiety and depression, which can affect cognitive function.

SUMMARY

Geriatric screening and assessment allows clinicians to care for older patients in an efficient, patient-centered manner. This framework includes standard screening questions that may trigger the use of standard geriatric assessment tools and/or other interventions. Additionally, it serves to complement the history and physical examination, and is critical for maximizing the health, function, safety, and quality of life of older patients.

REFERENCES

1. Kane RL, Ouslander JG, Resnick B, et al. Essentials of clinical geriatrics. 8th edition. New York: McGraw-Hill; 2018.
2. Seeman TE. Health promoting effects of friends and family on health outcomes in older adults. Am J Health Promot 2000;14(6):362–70.
3. Stroebe W. Social psychology and health. 2nd edition. Buckingham (England): Open University Press; 2000.
4. Lubben J, Blozik E, Gillmann G, et al. Performance of an abbreviated version of the Lubben Social Network Scale among three European community-dwelling older adult populations. Gerontologist 2006;46(4):503–13.
5. Khan N, Davis P, Wilkinson TJ, et al. Drinking patterns among older people in the community: hidden from medical attention? N Z Med J 2002;115(1148):72–5.
6. National Institute of Aging. When does drinking become a problem? 2017. Available at: https://www.nia.nih.gov/health/when-does-drinking-become-problem. Accessed June 6, 2018.
7. Draper B, Ridley N, Johnco C, et al. Screening for alcohol and substance use for older people in geriatric hospital and community health settings. Int Psychogeriatr 2015;27(1):157–66.
8. Philpot M, Pearson N, Petratou V, et al. Screening for problem drinking in older people referred to a mental health service: a comparison of CAGE and AUDIT. Aging Ment Health 2003;7(3):171–5.
9. Thomson MJ, Lietzau LK, Doty MM, et al. An analysis of elder abuse rates in Milwaukee County. WMJ 2011;110(6):271–6.
10. Yaffe MJ, Wolfson C, Lithwick M, et al. Development and validation of a tool to improve physician identification of elder abuse: the Elder Abuse Suspicion Index (EASI). J Elder Abuse Negl 2008;20(3):276–300.
11. Ramsaroop SD, Reid MC, Adelman RD. Completing an advance directive in the primary care setting: what do we need for success? J Am Geriatr Soc 2007;55(2): 277–83.
12. Reinhardt JP, Chichin E, Posner L, et al. Vital conversations with family in the nursing home: preparation for end-stage dementia care. J Soc Work End Life Palliat Care 2014;10(2):112–26.
13. Hing Wong A, Chin LE, Ping TL, et al. Clinical impact of education provision on determining advance care planning decisions among end stage renal disease patients receiving regular hemodialysis in University Malaya Medical Centre. Indian J Palliat Care 2016;22(4):437–45.
14. Hickman SE, Keevern E, Hammes BJ. Use of the physician orders for life-sustaining treatment program in the clinical setting: a systematic review of the literature. J Am Geriatr Soc 2015;63(2):341–50.
15. Reuben DB, Seeman TE, Keeler E, et al. Refining the categorization of physical functional status: the added value of combining self-reported and performance-based measures. J Gerontol A Biol Sci Med Sci 2004;59(10): 1056–61.
16. Reuben DB, Seeman TE, Keeler E, et al. The effect of self-reported and performance-based functional impairment on future hospital costs of community-dwelling older persons. Gerontologist 2004;44(3):401–7.
17. Graf C. The Lawton instrumental activities of daily living scale. Am J Nurs 2008; 108(4):52–62.
18. Lawton MP, Brody EM. Assessment of older people: self-maintaining and instrumental activities of daily living. Gerontologist 1969;9(3):179–86.

19. Katz S, Downs TD, Cash HR, et al. Progress in development of the index of ADL. Gerontologist 1970;10(1):20–30.

20. Katz S. Assessing self-maintenance: activities of daily living, mobility, and instrumental activities of daily living. J Am Geriatr Soc 1983;31:721–7.

21. Ouslander J, Reyes B. Clinical problems associated with the aging process. In: Jameson JL, Fauci AS, Kasper DL, et al, editors. Harrison's principles of internal medicine. 20th edition. McGraw-Hill Education/Medical, in press. Available at: http://accessmedicine.mhmedical.com/content.aspx?bookid=2129&sectionid=192535397. Accessed November 19, 2018.

22. American Geriatrics Society, Pomidor A. Clinician's guide to assessing and counseling older drivers. 3rd edition. Washington, DC: National Highway Traffic Safety Administration; 2016. Available at: https://www.nhtsa.gov/sites/nhtsa.dot.gov/files/812228_cliniciansguidetoolderdrivers.pdf. Accessed April 26, 2018.

23. Christ SL, Zheng DD, Swenor BK, et al. Longitudinal relationships among visual acuity, daily functional status, and mortality: the Salisbury Eye Evaluation study. JAMA Ophthalmol 2014;132:1400–6.

24. US Census Bureau. American Community Survey. 2013. Available at: http://aoa.acl.gov/Aging_Statistics/Profile/2014/index.aspx. Accessed November 4, 2017.

25. Reuben DB. Geriatric assessment. In: Goldman L, Schafer AI, editors. Goldman-Cecil medicine. 25th edition. Linn (MO): Elsevier; 2015. p. 102–6.

26. Reuben DB, Herr KA, Pacala JT, et al. Geriatrics at your fingertips. 19th edition. New York: The American Geriatrics Society; 2017. p. 4, 109, 138-9.

27. Final recommendation statement: hearing loss in older adults: screening. U.S. Preventive Services Task Force. 2016. Available at: https://www.uspreventiveservicestaskforce.org/Page/Document/RecommendationStatementFinal/hearing-loss-in-older-adults-screening. Accessed November 4, 2017.

28. Ventry IM, Weinstein B. The hearing handicap inventory for the elderly. A new tool. Ear Hear 1982;3:128–34.

29. Rochon PA, Gurwitz JH. The prescribing cascade revisited. Lancet 2017;389(10081):1778–80.

30. American Geriatrics Society 2015 Beers Criteria Update Expert Panel. American Geriatrics Society 2015 updated beers criteria for potentially inappropriate medication use in older adults. J Am Geriatr Soc 2015;63(11):2227–46.

31. Important facts about falls. Centers for Disease Control and Prevention; 2017. Available at: https://www.cdc.gov/homeandrecreationalsafety/falls/adultfalls.html. Accessed February 27, 2018.

32. STEADI - older adult fall prevention. Centers for Disease Control and Prevention; 2017. Available at: https://www.cdc.gov/steadi/index.html. Accessed February 27, 2018.

33. Ferrucci L, Studenski S. Clinical problems of aging. In: Kasper D, Fauci A, Hauser S, et al, editors. Harrison's principles of internal medicine. 19th edition. New York: McGraw-Hill; 2014. Available at: http://accessmedicine.mhmedical.com/content.aspx?bookid=1130&sectionid=66487220. Accessed April 25, 2018.

34. Brown JS, Bradley CS, Subak LL, et al. The sensitivity and specificity of a simple test to distinguish between urge and stress urinary incontinence. Ann Intern Med 2006;144(10):715–23.

35. Barry MJ, Fowler FJ, O'Leary MP, et al. The American Urological Association symptom index for benign prostatic hyperplasia. The Measurement Committee of the American Urological Association. J Urol 1992;148(5):1549–57.

36. Robertson RG, Jameson JL. Involuntary weight loss. In: Kasper D, Fauci A, Hauser S, et al, editors. Harrison's principles of internal medicine. 19th edition. New York: McGraw Hill; 2014. Available at: http://accessmedicine.mhmedical.com/content.aspx?bookid=1130&sectionid=79726329. Accessed April 25, 2018.

37. Czeisler CA, Scammell TE, Saper CB. Sleep disorders. In: Kasper D, Fauci A, Hauser S, et al, editors. Harrison's principles of internal medicine. 19th edition. New York: McGraw-Hill; 2014. Available at: http://accessmedicine.mhmedical.com/content.aspx?bookid=1130&sectionid=79725062. Accessed April 25, 2018.

38. Buysse DJ, Reynolds CF, Monk TH, et al. The Pittsburgh sleep quality index: a new instrument for psychiatric practice and research. Psychiatry Res 1989; 28(2):193–213.

39. Kroenke K, Spitzer RL, Williams JB. The patient health questionnaire-2: validity of a two-item depression screener. Med Care 2003;41:1284–92.

40. Kroenke K, Spitzer RL, Williams JB. The PHQ-9: validity of a brief depression severity measure. J Gen Intern Med 2001;16(9):606–13.

41. Sheikh JI, Yesavage JA. Geriatric depression scale (GDS): recent evidence and development of a shorter version. Clin Gerontol 1986;5(1–2):165–73.

42. Meehan PJ, Saltzman LE, Sattin RW. Suicides among older United States residents: epidemiologic characteristics and trends. Am J Public Health 1991; 81(9):1198–200.

43. Final recommendation statement: cognitive impairment in older adults: screening. U.S. Preventive Services Task Force; 2016. Available at: https://www.uspreventiveservicestaskforce.org/Page/Document/RecommendationStatementFinal/cognitive-impairment-in-older-adults-screening. Accessed November 4, 2017.

44. Inouye SK, van Dyck CH, Alessi CA, et al. Clarifying confusion: the confusion assessment method: a new method for detection of delirium. Ann Intern Med 1990;113:941–8.

45. Scanlan J, Borson S. The Mini-Cog: receiver operating characteristics with expert and naïve raters. Int J Geriatr Psychiatry 2001;16:216–22.

46. Nasreddine ZS, Phillips NA, Bédirian V, et al. The Montreal cognitive assessment, MoCA: a brief screening tool for mild cognitive impairment. J Am Geriatr Soc 2005;53:695–9.

47. Tariq SH, Tumosa N, Chibnall JT, et al. Comparison of the Saint Louis University mental status examination and the mini-mental state examination for detecting dementia and mild neurocognitive disorder - a pilot study. Am J Geriatr Psychiatry 2006;14:900–10.

48. Folstein MF, Folstein SE, McHugh PR. Mini-mental state: a practical method for grading the cognitive state of patients for the clinician. J Psychiatr Res 1975; 12:189–98.

49. The Gerontological Society of America. Kickstart, assess, evaluate, and refer toolkit: 4- step process to detecting cognitive impairment and earlier diagnosis of dementia: approaches and tools for primary care providers. 2017. Available at: https://www.geron.org/images/gsa/kaer/gsa-kaer-toolkit.pdf. Accessed November 4, 2017.

Breast Cancer Screening
Why Can't Everyone Agree?

Veronica Jordan, MD, MS[a],*, Muneeza Khan, MD[b], Donna Prill, MD[c]

KEYWORDS

- Breast cancer • Screening • Mammography • Clinical breast examination
- Self breast examination • BRCA1/2 • Shared decision making

KEY POINTS

- Mammography is the only screening modality known to reduce breast cancer mortality.
- All women aged 50 to 74 should have at least biennial screening mammography.
- Younger women (less than 50) and older women (greater than 74) should participate in shared decision making with their primary care physicians regarding the risks and benefits of earlier initiation or later termination of screening.
- Shared decision making should include an assessment of the woman's individual risk for breast cancer and her vulnerability to the risks of increased screening, including false positives as well as potential for overdiagnosis and overtreatment.
- Neither clinical breast examination nor self breast examination has been shown to improve rates of breast cancer detection, prognosis, or breast cancer–related mortality.

CLINICAL DESCRIPTION OF DISEASE
Overview

Breast cancer is a disease that results in the uncontrolled proliferation of malignant cells in the breast. This process can start anywhere in the lobules, ducts, or stromal tissue of the breast and then gives rise to various types of breast cancer.

Symptoms

Most early breast cancers are asymptomatic and discovered on screening mammography.
Typical symptoms of breast cancer include the following:

- Breast swelling
- Fixed, firm lumps or bumps with irregular borders

Disclosure: The authors have nothing to disclose.
[a] Santa Rosa Family Medicine Residency, 3569 Round Barn Circle, Suite 200, Santa Rosa, CA 95403, USA; [b] Saint Francis Family Medicine Residency, 1301 Primacy Parkway, Memphis, TN 38119, USA; [c] Research Family Medicine Residency, 6675 Holmes Road, Suite 450, Kansas City, MO 64131, USA
* Corresponding author.
E-mail address: veronica.a.jordan@gmail.com

Prim Care Clin Office Pract 46 (2019) 97–115
https://doi.org/10.1016/j.pop.2018.10.010
0095-4543/19/© 2018 Elsevier Inc. All rights reserved.

- Overlying skin changes, such as thickening, discoloration, dimpling, or irritation
- Nipple discharge or retraction
- Pain in the breast or nipple

Risk Factors

Risk factors for breast cancer are listed in **Table 1**. Identifying a woman's individual risk factors allows physicians to risk-stratify patients and engage in shared decision making regarding specific screening recommendations; it also allows physicians counsel women on modifiable risk factors and important lifestyle changes.

Hormonal factors

Most breast cancers require a hormonal stimulus over a long duration of time to proliferate; this explains why being a woman and aging are the 2 most important risk factors for developing breast cancer.[1] Early menarche (before age 12) and late menopause (after age 55) increase a woman's risk, likely because of prolonged lifetime estrogen exposure.[2] Exposure to estrogen through postmenopausal hormone replacement therapy (HRT) longer than 5 years (risk is increased with the addition of progesterone) also increases the risk of developing breast cancer.[3] Being overweight or obese is also considered a risk factor.[4]

Prolonged use of combined oral contraceptives (OCPs) increases a woman's lifetime risk of breast cancer[5]; however, OCPs substantially reduce the risk of ovarian, endometrial, and colorectal cancer. Using OCPs for at least 5 years may contribute to a slight decrease in the total risk of cancer. These medications provide effective birth control as well as treatment of menorrhagia and dysmenorrhea. Thus, the risks and benefits must be weighed when considering the use of OCPs, especially because the absolute increase in risk of developing breast cancer is small.[6]

Table 1 Risk factors for breast cancer	
Gender	Female
Aging	>50 y
Genetics	BRCA1 and BRCA2 mutations
Personal history of breast cancer	Higher likelihood of recurrence
Family history of breast cancer	First-degree female or male relative, multiple family members
Reproductive	Menarche before age 12 Menopause after age 55 Nulliparity Late age of first pregnancy (after age 30)
Hormonal: OCP, HRT	OCP: Current or recent use HRT exposure longer than 5 y
Lifestyle	Obesity Sedentary lifestyle Alcohol consumption (>1 drink per day)
Dense breast tissue	More tissue can obscure lesions on mammography
History of benign breast disease	Proliferative lesions such as atypical hyperplasia or lobular carcinoma in situ
Radiation	Chest/breast exposure to radiation at young age
DES exposure	DES
Smoking, chemicals, nightshift work	May increase risk

Additional risk factors for breast cancer include nulliparity or late (after age 30) pregnancy,[2] physical inactivity,[7] having dense breasts,[8] personal or family history of breast cancer,[9] history of noncancerous breast abnormalities with proliferative patterns,[10] history of radiation to the chest or breast before age 30,[11] drinking more than one alcoholic drink per day,[12] and diethylstilbestrol (DES) exposure.[13]

Heredity/genetics
In the United States, only between 5% and 10% of breast cancers in women are hereditary, meaning that the breast cancer is related to a known genetic mutation.[14] Approximately 6% of male breast cancers are due to BRCA2 mutations.[15] Hereditary breast and ovarian cancer syndrome is most commonly caused by mutations in BRCA1 and BRCA2, genes that code for a DNA repair pathway important in tumor suppression. The loss of either gene confers a higher risk of breast cancer as well as other cancers.

Environmental and chemical exposure
There are emerging data that environmental and chemical exposures play a role in breast cancer risk with particular concern regarding exposure during breast development to dichlorodiphenyltrichloroethane, dioxins, perfluorooctane-sulfonamide, and air pollution.[16,17] There remains controversy as to how nightshift work may or may not contribute to higher risks of breast cancer.[18]

Epidemiology

Incidence
Breast cancer is the most common non–skin cancer in US women with an incidence of 123.9 per 100,000 women.[19] About 12.4% of women (1 in 8) will develop breast cancer at some point in their lives.[20] Annually, there are an estimated 237,000 new cases and 41,000 deaths due to female breast cancer.[21] Incidence of female breast cancer increases after age 25 and peaks in the 70- to 74-year range at 461.9 per 100,000 cases (**Fig. 1**).[22]

Between 1975 and 2015, breast cancer mortality declined from 31.4 to 20.3 deaths per 100,000 women.[23] This decrease in mortality has been attributed to a combination of increased mammographic screening and improved treatments.[24] However, breast cancer still remains the second leading cause of cancer death in US women.[1]

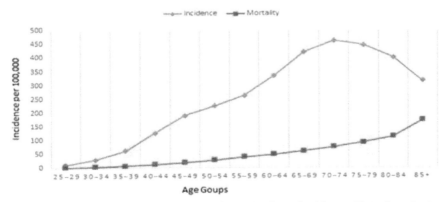

Fig. 1. Breast cancer incidence and mortality by age in the United States. (*Data from* Centers for Disease Control and Prevention. United States cancer statistics: data visualizations. Available at: https://gis.cdc.gov/cancer/USCS/DataViz.html. Accessed July 3, 2018.)

Racial and ethnic disparities

White women are slightly more likely to be diagnosed with breast cancer than African American, Hispanic, or Asian women. However, African American women are more likely to be diagnosed with more aggressive and advanced breast cancer at a younger age.[25] African American women have a higher mortality of 27.6 per 100,000 women (compared with 19.8 for white women; **Fig. 2**).[22] Reasons for this are not completely understood, although contributing factors include low socioeconomic status, differential access to health care, and probable disease-related molecular differences.[26,27]

Screening recommendations

Key considerations when developing screening recommendations include the following:

1. The prevalence of disease in the screened population
2. The effectiveness or benefit of the screening procedure (eg, reduction in breast-cancer mortality, all-cause mortality)
3. Any potential risks and cost of screening (eg, false positives [FPs], overdiagnosis)

The answers to these questions lead experts to determine which modalities to recommend as screening tools for a particular disease (eg, mammogram vs clinical breast examination [CBE] vs self breast examination [SBE] vs MRI). Once the modality is established, more specific questions follow; this is where breast cancer screening gets controversial:

- Which modalities should be used?
- When should screening begin and end?
- What is the appropriate interval for screening?
- What are the benefits and risks of screening?

Screening Modalities

Self breast examinations

SBEs were previously considered to be an essential component of breast cancer screening. Two randomized control trials (RCTs) evaluated the role of SBE as a breast

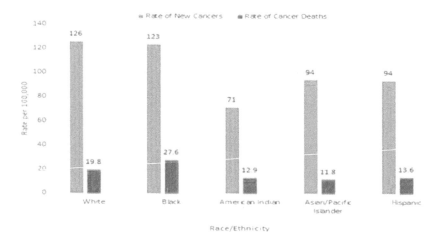

Fig. 2. Rates of female breast cancer incidence and mortality by race/ethnicity. (*Data from* Centers for Disease Control and Prevention. United States cancer statistics: data visualizations. Available at: https://gis.cdc.gov/cancer/USCS/DataViz.html. Accessed July 3, 2018.)

cancer screening modality: one in China with 267,000 female factory workers[28] and one in Russia with more than 193,000 women.[29] Both RCTs failed to show a breast cancer mortality benefit due to SBE.

The Chinese study found equal numbers of breast cancer in both groups with no significant difference in staging at time of detection. The Russian study demonstrated earlier detection of breast cancer in the SBE group compared with the control group with significantly improved 15-year survival, but overall breast cancer mortality remained unaffected.[23] In both studies, SBE led to an increased number of unnecessary biopsies for benign breast lesions.

The US Preventive Services Task Force (USPSTF), American Academy of Family Physicians (AAFP), and Canadian Preventive Task Force currently recommend against SBE. The American Cancer Society (ACS) recommends counseling regarding benefits and limitations of SBE. The American College of Obstetrics and Gynecology (ACOG) and National Comprehensive Cancer network recommend breast self-awareness.

Of note, there is no standardized definition of "breast self-awareness," and there have been no studies to date on the impact of breast self-awareness on breast cancer outcomes. It has been argued that recommending breast self-awareness might actually be harmful to women in the same ways SBE has been shown to be harmful by increasing unnecessary testing and biopsies without improving outcomes.[30]

Clinical breast examinations

Many physicians continue to perform CBE,[31] although their role in breast cancer screening remains controversial.[32] An ideal screening test should be exquisitely sensitive and specific. Studies show that CBE has a high specificity (94%–99%) but a very low sensitivity (21%–54%),[33–35] which means that although the presence of a palpable mass on CBE is a good predictor of breast cancer, the absence of a mass is less reassuring. In other words, a normal CBE does not exclude the presence of breast cancer.

Anecdotal evidence and retrospective studies do support a role for CBE, particularly in more aggressive cancers,[36–38] but there have been very few RCTs designed to evaluate its benefit as a screening tool. One poorly designed study in the Philippines was discontinued after only one round because of poor community acceptance.[39] Two more are still in process in Egypt[40] and India.[41]

Thus, the best data to evaluate the efficacy of CBE are observational and/or in conjunction with mammography. The most influential negative study was a Canadian RCT of 39,405 women aged 50 to 59 years, comparing CBE versus CBE plus mammogram screening with 13 years of follow-up. There was no difference in mortalities within both groups, concluding that there was no added benefit of CBE over screening mammogram.[42]

As such, the AAFP and the USPSTF found insufficient evidence to recommend for or against CBE. ACOG, ACS, National Comprehensive Cancer Network (NCCN), and Canadian Preventive Task Force recommend a range of CBE options, starting as early as age 20, every 1 to 3 years (**Table 2**). There may be a larger role for CBE in developing countries where women have limited access to mammography.[43]

Mammography

Mammography is the only screening modality that has shown a reduction in breast cancer mortality.[44] To date, at least 9 separate RCTs, with more than 600,000 women, were conducted in Canada, the United States, the United Kingdom, Russia, and Sweden. All of them showed reduction in breast cancer–related mortality using screening mammography.[44] There is no evidence that screening mammography reduces all-cause mortality.

Table 2
Comparison of breast cancer screening recommendations

Screening Modality	US Preventive Services Task Force	American Academy of Family Physicians	American Cancer Society	American College of Obstetrics and Gynecology	American College of Radiology	National Comprehensive Cancer Network	Canadian Task Force on Preventive Health Care
SBEs	Recommend against	Recommend against	Counsel about benefits and limitations	Breast self-awareness encouraged	None	Breast self-awareness encouraged	Recommend against
CBEs	Insufficient evidence	Insufficient evidence	Every 3 y from 20–39 y of age and annually thereafter	Every 1–3 y from 20–39 y and annually thereafter	None	Insufficient evidence	Every 1–2 y beginning at 40 y
Mammography	Biennial screening for women 50–74 y	Biennial screening for women 50–74 y	Annual screening beginning at 45 y, then, biennial beginning at 55 y	Annual OR biennial screening for women beginning at 40 y	Annual screening beginning at 40 y	Annual screening beginning at 40 y	Screening every 2–3 y beginning at 50 y, through 74 y
MRI	Insufficient evidence	Insufficient evidence	Offer annually to women at high risk	Offer annually to women at high risk	None	Offer annually to women at high risk	None

Each of these RCTs was slightly different: each enrolled women at different ages, compared different screening intervals, randomized differently, and tracked the breast cancer cases and deaths differently.[45] All of these variables contributed to differences in outcomes, effect size, interpretations, and ultimately, different recommendations (see **Table 2**). Most studies were also done before many of the current breast cancer treatment strategies were in place, which means they may overestimate mortality benefit.

Interval for routine mammography

There are no head-to-head trials comparing the risks versus benefits of different screening intervals. The range of screening intervals in the RCTs used to inform current recommendations is 12 to 36 months; in some cases, the interval varied by age groups even within the same RCT. Per the USPSTF 2016 Systematic Review, the existing trials do not provide enough information to analyze the specific effect of different screening intervals.[45]

Observational studies might help with the understanding of the effect of screening intervals on breast cancer outcomes. For example, in Canada, routine screening changed from annual screening for all women aged 40 to 74 to biennial for 50 to 74 and annual only for women aged 40 to 49 years. After this change, there was no difference in breast cancer mortality in any age group.[46] An observational study in Finland showed no difference between annual and triennial screening in women aged 40 to 49.[47]

Age for initiating and ending routine screening mammography

US Preventive Services Task Force (2016) The USPSTF recommends biennial mammogram screenings (every other year) for women aged 50 to 74 (B). For women aged 40 to 49, the decision to start screening should be an individual one. Women who feel that the risk is less than the benefit may choose to start screening biennially (C). For women greater than 75, the USPSTF concludes there is insufficient evidence to recommend for or against mammogram screening (I) (**Table 3**).

The women most likely to benefit from screening are those between the ages of 60 and 69. They acknowledge that for women aged 40 to 49, screening mammography reduces risk of breast cancer death, but the number of FPs and biopsies is larger (see later discussion for more in-depth discussion). As women move into their later 40s, the balance between benefit and risk likely improves. Women with a first-degree relative (mother, sister, child) are at higher risk and may benefit from earlier screening.

The AAFP has endorsed the USPSTF recommendations.[48] Other professional US organizations disagree with the USPSTF and continue to recommend earlier and more frequent screening.

The American Cancer Society (2015) In 2015, the ACS updated their 2003 breast cancer screening guidelines, recommending that women with an average risk of breast cancer start annual mammograms at age 45 with the option to decrease frequency to every other year starting at age 55 (or continuing annually, if they prefer).[49] They define women with an "average risk" as all women except those with a personal history of breast cancer, those with a known genetic mutation (eg, BRCA), or those who have received chest radiation at a young age.

In addition, the ACS recommends that women may choose to start mammograms as early as age 40, and they should continue to be screened for breast cancer as long as they are in reasonable health with at least a 10-year life expectancy.

Table 3
US Preventive Services Task Force grade definitions

Grade	Definition	Suggestions for Practice
A	The USPSTF recommends the service; there is high certainty that the net benefit is substantial	Offer or provide this service
B	The USPSTF recommends the service; there is high certainty that the net benefit is moderate or there is moderate certainty that the net benefit is moderate to substantial	Offer or provide this service
C	The USPSTF recommends selectively offering or providing this service to individual patients based on professional judgment and patient preferences; there is at least moderate certainty that the net benefit is small	Offer or provide this service for selected patients depending on individual circumstances
D	The USPSTF recommends against the service; there is moderate or high certainty that the service has no net benefit or that the harms outweigh the benefits	Discourage the use of this service
I	The USPSTF concludes that the current evidence is insufficient to assess the balance of benefits and harms of the service; evidence is lacking, of poor quality, or conflicting, and the balance of benefits and harms cannot be determined	Read the clinical considerations section of USPSTF Recommendation Statement; if the service is offered, patients should understand the uncertainty about the balance of benefits and harms

From U.S. Preventive Services Task Force. USPSTF grade definitions after 2012. Available at: https://www.uspreventiveservicestaskforce.org/Page/Name/grade-definitions. Accessed July 3, 2018; with permission.

The ACS does not recommend CBEs for breast cancer screening in women at average risk.

In their recommendation statement, ACS advocates for starting mammogram screening at age 45 (rather than 40 or 50) predicated on their position that 10-year intervals used in much of the literature are historic and artificial, based on study design rather than evidence. Breast cancer incidence increases with age, and the ACS proposes that a 45-year-old woman's absolute risk of breast cancer and dying from breast cancer is more similar to a 50 year old than a 40 year old, and that the screening intervals should reflect this (**Table 4**).

Table 4
Breast cancer statistics in 5-y intervals (ages 40–54)

Age (y)	5-y Absolute Risk of Breast Cancer (%)	Incident Breast Cancers in the Population (%)	Breast Cancer Deaths by Age at Diagnosis (%)
40–44	0.6	6	7
45–49	0.9	10	10
50–54	1.1	12	11

Data from Oeffinger KC, Fontham ET, Etzioni R, et al. Breast cancer screening for women at average risk 2015 guideline update from the American Cancer Society. JAMA 2015;314(15):1599–614.

The ACS also recommends that there is enough evidence for increased benefit of annual (vs biennial) mammography in younger women to justify the increased risk of FPs that occur with more frequent screening through age 55.

The American College of Obstetricians and Gynecologists (2017) In 2017, the ACOG released their updated breast cancer screening recommendations.[50] The ACOG continues to recommend that women be offered screening mammography starting at age 40; they advocate for shared decision making and recommend that for women who choose not to start at 40, they should start screening "no later than age 50."

The ACOG recommends that women of average risk should have mammogram every 1 to 2 years, with the interval based on shared decision making. Finally, they recommend that women should continue screening at least until age 75 and that continued screening thereafter should also be a shared decision-making process.

The American College of Radiology (2017/2018) In 2017 and 2018, The American College of Radiology (ACR) released updated screening recommendations, which propose a risk assessment at age 30 to determine whether a woman should start mammograms before age 40. They continue to recommend that average-risk women start screening at age 40 and continue annually until at least 75 years of age.[51]

The ACR makes specific screening recommendations for African American women (who they identify as being higher risk) and recommend that women of higher risk and with a history of breast cancer before 50 be screened by MRI.[52]

International recommendations A recent review of cancer screening recommendations in 21 high-income countries (mostly Europe and North America) found that the recommendations for breast cancer screening are quite similar internationally[53] with 50 to 69 being the most common screening age range, although several other countries increase screening to the age of 74. Most European countries recommend a 2-year screening interval (the United Kingdom recommends every 3 years). The ACR has the longest age range of any organization and is the only organization in the world still recommending annual screening.

Benefits of Routine Mammography Screening

Reduction in breast cancer mortality

It is difficult to extrapolate the actual reduction in breast cancer mortality due to screening mammography from available data. The effect varies based on a woman's baseline risk, age at screening, frequency of screening, follow-up, and methods used to make the estimates. A meta-analysis of 9 RCTs on screening mammography shows a relative risk reduction that ranges from 0.67 to 0.90 for women aged 60 to 69 and 70 to 74, respectively,[45] which translates to a 10% to 33% decreased risk of dying from breast cancer for women who receive screening mammography. The combined risk reduction for women aged 50 to 69 years is 0.78 (or 22%). Breast cancer mortality reduction reported by decade is displayed in **Fig. 3**.

Results from these same data were used to estimate the absolute mortality reduction based on women invited to be screened. The number of deaths prevented by age group (per 10,000 women screened for 10 years) is reported in **Table 5**.

In addition to RCTs, there have also been systematic reviews of observational data from population-based screening programs in Europe and the United Kingdom of women aged 50 to 69 attempting to estimate the mortality benefit of screening mammography.[54] These observational studies, which evaluated outcomes before

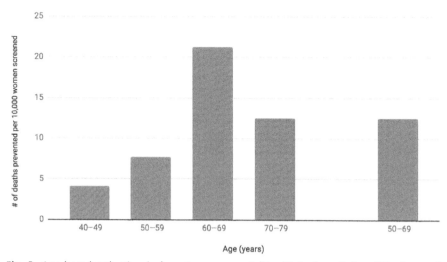

Fig. 3. Age-based reduction in breast cancer mortality. (*Data from* Nelson HD, Cantor A, Humphrey L, et al. Screening for breast cancer: a systematic review to update the 2009 U.S. Preventive Services Task Force recommendation. Rockville (MD): Agency for Healthcare Research and Quality; 2016. (Evidence Syntheses, No. 124.) 3.)

and after implementation of nationwide screening programs, found a mortality benefit ranging from 28% to 35%.[55–57]

Harms of Routine Mammography Screening

False positives (FP)

An FP is a screening test that is abnormal (positive test) but that is ultimately found to be normal (without disease) upon follow-up diagnostic testing.

The rate of FP with mammogram screening in women who start screening at age 40 and are screened annually for 10 years has been estimated to be 61.3% if screened annually versus 41.6% if screened biennially (**Fig. 4**).[58] Most of these are corrected after a follow-up diagnostic mammogram or ultrasound. The rate of an FP that will lead

Table 5			
Breast cancer mortality reduction, by age			
Age (y)	**No. of Trials**	**Risk Reduction (RR), Confidence Interval (CI)**	**No. of Deaths Prevented per 10,000 Women Screened for 10 y**
40–49	9	0.88 CI (0.73–1.03)	4.1
50–59	7	0.86 CI (0.68–0.97)	7.7
60–69	5	0.67 CI (0.54–0.83)	21.3
70–79	3	0.90 CI (0.51–1.28)	12.5
50–69[a]	5	0.78	12.5

[a] This age range is a separate estimated absolute mortality reduction in the usual screening interval.

Data from Nelson HD, Cantor A, Humphrey L, et al. Screening for breast cancer: a systematic review to update the 2009 U.S. Preventive Services Task Force recommendation. Rockville (MD): Agency for Healthcare Research and Quality; 2016. (Evidence Syntheses, No. 124.) 3.

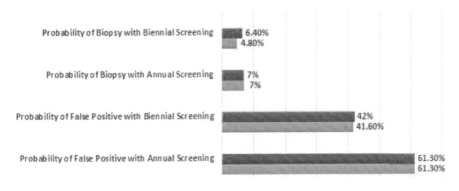

■ Age 50–59 ▨ Age 40–49

Fig. 4. Cumulative probability of FP after 10 years of mammograms. (*Data from* Hubbard RA, Kerlikowske K, Flowers CI, et al. Cumulative probability of false-positive recall or biopsy recommendation after 10 years of screening mammography: a cohort study. Ann Intern Med 2011;155(8):481–92.)

to an unnecessary biopsy is also increased with more frequent screening: 7% versus 4.8% (annual vs biennial).

Of note, family history of breast cancer, high breast density, and previous benign breast biopsy are associated with higher rates of FP and false-negative results across all age groups. Premenopausal status, use of menopausal HRT, and lower body mass index (BMI) may also increase risk of FP but in specific age groups only.

Rates of FP results and biopsy are highest among women receiving annual mammography, those with heterogeneously dense or extremely dense breasts, and those either 40 to 49 years old or who used combination HRT.

Overdiagnosis

Overdiagnosis is the concept that some percentage of screen-detected cancers would not have led to symptomatic cancer if they had not been detected in the first place. Overdiagnosis is considered the most important harm of screening because it would lead to unnecessary treatment. It is perhaps the most challenging phenomenon to measure and/or predict without natural history studies, which are hard to come by in an era when women are always offered treatment for breast cancer. No published study directly provides a reliable estimate of overdiagnosis.

For every case of invasive breast cancer detected by mammography screening in women aged 40 to 49 years, 464 women had screening mammography, 58 were recommended for additional imaging, and 10 were recommended for biopsies. These estimates declined with age. Unadjusted estimates from 13 observational studies included in the Euroscreen review indicated overdiagnosis rates ranging from 0% to 54%.[45] For 6 studies that adjusted overdiagnosis estimates for breast cancer risk and lead time, rates varied from 1% to 10%.

Anxiety and distress

Women with FP results have more anxiety, psychological distress, and breast cancer–specific worry after screening compared with those with normal screening results in most studies. Anxiety improved over time for most women, but persisted for more than 2 years for some.[45]

Radiation exposure
Models calculate the number of deaths due to radiation-induced cancer using estimates for digital mammography is between 2 per 100,000 in women aged 50 to 59 years screened biennially and up to 11 per 100,000 in women ages 40 to 59 years screened annually.[45]

Pain during procedure
Although many women may experience pain during mammography (1% to 77%), the proportion of those experiencing pain who do not attend future screening varies (11% to 46%).[45] It is unclear how much pain is a barrier for future mammogram.

Special Considerations

Dense breasts
Breast density refers to the amount of fibroglandular tissue relative to fat in the breasts and increased breast density results in more opaque areas on the mammogram; it is not based on how the breasts feel on palpation during SBE or CBE.[59] Women with increased breast density have a higher lifetime risk of breast cancer. Increased density also decreases the sensitivity and specificity of mammography.[60]

There is no gold standard for breast density measurement, and although descriptive categories have been established, the assessment of breast density is ultimately subjective and based on visual estimation of the radiologist.[60] The BI-RADS (Breast Imaging Reporting and Database System) includes an assessment of breast tissue composition, organized into 4 categories:

a. Almost entirely fatty
b. Scattered areas of fibroglandular density
c. Heterogeneously dense, may obscure small masses
d. Extremely dense, lowers the sensitivity of mammography

It is estimated that 43% of US women aged 40 to 70 have "dense breasts" (category c or d); associated factors include younger age, use of HRT, and lower BMI.[61]

Because of the increased risk of breast cancer and decreased sensitivity of mammography to detect cancer, alternate or supplemental breast cancer screening methods have been proposed. These methods include more frequent mammography,[60] supplemental ultrasound,[62,63] MRI, and digital breast tomosynthesis (DBT) (ie, 3D mammography). Data are mixed for each of these modalities because although they may detect additional breast cancers, they do so at the risk of increased FPs, and results are not reliably reproducible.[64]

As such, no medical organization currently recommends supplementary screening on the basis of breast density alone; the USPSTF has found insufficient evidence to recommend any particular kind of additional testing specifically for women with dense breasts.[65]

Currently, state-specific legislation mandates that women with dense breasts on mammography be notified of the finding and encourages supplementary testing irrespective of the risk of breast cancer.[66]

Women with greater than 20% lifetime risk
The USPSTF and AAFP currently do not recommend supplemental or alternative screening for higher-risk women. However, ACOG, ACS, NCCN, and ACR recommend annual supplementary MRI for women with greater than 20% lifetime risk of breast cancer. This high-risk group primarily includes women with genetic mutations, but also those with a history of chest radiation or lobular carcinoma in situ, and women with enough cumulative risk factors to meet the risk threshold.

Numerous online breast cancer risk assessment tools exist and may be used to assist clinicians and women in estimating their lifetime risk and guide decision making. A few examples follow:

https://www.cancer.gov/bcrisktool/
https://www.assessyourrisk.org/
https://www.mdcalc.com/gail-model-breast-cancer-risk
https://breastcancerrisk.canceraustralia.gov.au/
https://tools.bcsc-scc.org/bc5yearrisk/calculator.html

These interactive tools use a woman's family history and take into account various other risk factors to estimate her lifetime risk of developing breast cancer. Based on which factors are taken into account, each of these tools may potentially underestimate or overestimate breast cancer risk. Different tools may generate very different results for the same woman. Such limitations in accuracy must be taken into consideration during the decision-making process.

Preventive Recommendations

Average-risk women

For average-risk women, breast cancer prevention recommendations reflect the following known modifiable risk factors:

- Do not smoke
- Be physically active
- Avoid or limit alcohol (less than 1 drink per day)
- Keep a healthy weight
- Breastfeed
- Limit dose and duration of HRT
- Avoid exposure to radiation and environmental pollution

High-risk women (genetics)

The USPSTF recommends that primary care providers screen women who have family members with breast, ovarian, tubal, or peritoneal cancer with 1 of several screening tools regarding their family history. These tools (see later discussion) are designed to identify women with an increased risk for potentially harmful mutations in BRCA1 or BRCA2. Per the USPSTF recommendation, women who screen positive should be referred to genetic counseling, and, if indicated after counseling, have BRCA testing. The USPSTF recommends that this screening be initiated when a woman turns consenting age (18 years old) and be revisited periodically (every 5–10 years) by primary care clinicians.

Family history screening tool There are several tools the USPSTF recommends that can be used to assess a woman's risk for hereditary breast cancer, as follows:

- The Ontario Family History Tool Assessment
- Manchester Scoring System
- Referral Screening Tool
- Pedigree Assessment Tool
- Family history screening-7 (FHS-7)

The FHS-7 (**Box 1**) and The Referral Screening Tool (found at www.breastcancergenescreen.org) are the simplest to administer. Note that these tools help primary care physicians to know when to refer to genetic counselor, not whether to order BRCA testing.

Box 1
Family history screening-7

1. Did any of your first-degree relatives have breast or ovarian cancer?

2. Did any of your relatives have bilateral breast cancer?

3. Did any man in your family have breast cancer?

4. Did any woman in your family have breast and ovarian cancer?

5. Did any woman in your family have breast cancer before the age of 50 years?

6. Do you have 2 or more relatives with breast and/or ovarian cancer?

7. Do you have 2 or more relatives with breast and/or bowel cancer?

Refer to genetic counseling with one or more positive response.
From Ashton-Prolla P, Giacomazzi J, Schmidt AV, et al. Development and validation of a simple questionnaire for the identification of hereditary breast cancer in primary care. BMC Cancer 2009;283.

BRCA mutation carriers

For high-risk women who test positive for BRCA1/2, potential recommendations include earlier and more frequent screening, surgery (prophylactic mastectomy and salpingo-oophorectomy), chemoprevention (antiestrogen medications, eg, tamoxifen and raloxifene), and lifestyle measures.[67] Lifestyle measures include breastfeeding, maintaining a normal body weight, limiting alcohol use, and avoiding HRT. The decision to proceed with any of these options should, if possible, be done in consultation with high-risk follow-up clinics that specifically focus on screening of individuals with known hereditary cancer syndrome.

Shared Decision Making

Shared decision making is an important component of patient-centered care. This process enables clinicians and patients to work together when making test or treatment decisions based on evidence that balances risks and expected outcomes with the patient's personal goals, preferences, and values. Shared decision making is especially important in complex situations whereby there is more than one reasonable option and no single "right" answer. It encourages a strong patient-physician bond and empowers the patient to take an active role in their health management.

Shared decision making requires the clinician do some work understanding the unique perspective and needs of the individual patient; it also often means homework for the patient, like reading materials, DVDs, and patient decision aids.

RCTs consistently demonstrate the effectiveness of patient decision aids. A 2011 Cochrane Review found that compared with controls, patients who used decision aids had increased knowledge, more accurate risk perceptions, reduced internal conflict about decisions, and a greater likelihood of receiving care aligned with their values. Moreover, fewer patients were undecided or passive in the decision-making process: changes that are essential for patients' adherence to therapies.[68]

SUMMARY

Although essentially every professional organization in the world agrees that women aged 50 to 74 should get screening mammograms to reduce the risk of dying from breast cancer, there is still much to debate regarding the younger and older age groups as well as in the screening interval for all age groups. Supplemental screening is also controversial.

These debates have led to a range of differing and evolving recommendations, which are confusing for both patients and clinicians. There is no clear line in which breast cancer incidence, mortality benefit, and risk of screening perfectly coincide. Therefore, in some ways, any line drawn is somewhat arbitrary.

In summary,

- Although breast cancer is less common in younger women, the incidence is not zero. By not screening younger women, it is accepted that some breast cancers will be missed.
- If one chooses to screen younger women and/or screen at more frequent intervals, it is accepted that there are real risks associated with screening, namely more FPs and the possibility of overdiagnosis and overtreatment.
- Estimates of the benefit of discovering breast cancer at a range of ages differ widely, and this discrepancy leads to a different assessment of risk and benefit.
- The recommended ages for screening have been drawn historically in 10-year increments, based more on how RCTs have been designed than on natural history of the disease. The new ACS recommendations challenge that notion and push us to question the limitations of old perspectives.
- Alternative and supplemental screening modalities like DBT and MRI may pick up breast cancers that were missed on mammography but the cost-benefit ratio and risks are not well delineated.
- Risk assessment tools are evolving to help primary care physicians do this better, but there is much work to be done.
- Shared decision making enables a physicians and patient partnership when deciding on which test or treatment is best for the patient.

REFERENCES

1. Steiner E, Klubert D, Knutson D. Assessing breast cancer risk in women. Am Fam Physician 2008;78(12):1361–6.
2. Kelsey JL, Gammon MD, John EM. Reproductive factors and breast cancer. Epidemiol Rev 1993;15(1):36–47.
3. Collins JA, Blake JM, Crosignani PG. Breast cancer risk with postmenopausal hormonal treatment. Hum Reprod Update 2005;11(6):545–60.
4. Bernstein L. Epidemiology of endocrine-related risk factors for breast cancer. J Mammary Gland Biol Neoplasia 2002;7(1):3–15.
5. Gierisch JM, Coeytaux RR, Urrutia RP, et al. Oral contraceptive use and risk of breast, cervical, colorectal, and endometrial cancers: a systematic review. Cancer Epidemiol Biomarkers Prev 2013;22(11):1931–43.
6. Mørch LS, Skovlund CW, Hannaford PC, et al. Contemporary hormonal contraception and the risk of breast cancer. N Engl J Med 2017;377:2228–39.
7. Steindorf K, Ritte R, Eomois PP, et al. Physical activity and risk of breast cancer overall and by hormone receptor status: the European prospective investigation into cancer and nutrition. Int J Cancer 2013;132(7):1667–78.
8. Boyd NF, Guo H, Martin LJ, et al. Mammographic density and the risk and detection of breast cancer. N Engl J Med 2007;356(3):227–36.
9. Singletary SE. Rating the risk factors for breast cancer. Ann Surg 2003;237:474–82.
10. Hartmann LC, Sellers TA, Frost MH, et al. Benign breast disease and the risk of breast cancer. N Engl J Med 2005;353(3):229–37.

11. Laden F, Hunter DJ. Environmental risk factors and female breast cancer. Annu Rev Public Health 1998;19:101–23.
12. Hamajima N, Hirose K, Tajima K, et al, for the Collaborative Group on Hormonal Factors in Breast Cancer. Alcohol, tobacco and breast cancer—collaborative re-analysis of individual data from 53 epidemiological studies, including 58,515 women with breast cancer and 95,067 women without the disease. Br J Cancer 2002;87(11):1234–45.
13. Colton T, Greenberg ER, Noller K, et al. Breast cancer in mothers prescribed diethylstilbestrol in pregnancy. Further follow-up. JAMA 1993;269(16):2096–100.
14. American Cancer Society. Breast cancer facts & figures 2015-2016. Atlanta (GA): American Cancer Society, Inc.; 2015.
15. American Cancer Society. Risk factors for breast cancer in men. Available at: https://www.cancer.org/cancer/breast-cancer-in-men/causes-risks-prevention/risk-factors.html. Accessed July 1, 2018.
16. Gray JM, Rasanayagam S, Engel C, et al. State of the evidence 2017: an update on the connection between breast cancer and the environment. Environ Health 2017;16(1):94.
17. Rodgers KM, Udesky JO, Rudel RA, et al. Environmental chemicals and breast cancer: an updated review of epidemiological literature informed by biological mechanisms. Environ Res 2018;160:152–82.
18. Jia Y, Lu Y, Wu K, et al. Does night work increase the risk of breast cancer? A systematic review and meta-analysis of epidemiological studies. Cancer Epidemiol 2013;37(3):197–206.
19. U.S. Cancer Statistics Working Group. United States cancer statistics: 1999–2014 incidence and mortality web-based report. Atlanta (GA): Department of Health and Human Services, Centers for Disease Control and Prevention, and National Cancer Institute; 2017. Available at: http://www.cdc.gov/uscs.
20. Howlader N, Noone AM, Krapcho M, et al, editors. SEER cancer statistics review, 1975–2009 (Vintage 2009 Populations). Bethesda (MD): National Cancer Institute; 2012.
21. CDC basic information about breast cancer. Available at: https://www.cdc.gov/cancer/breast/basic_info/index.htm. Accessed July 3, 2018.
22. CDC United States Cancer Statistics:Data Visualizations. Available at: https://gis.cdc.gov/cancer/USCS/DataViz.html. Accessed July 3, 2018.
23. National Cancer Institute. Available at: https://seer.cancer.gov/statfacts/html/breast.html. Accessed July 3, 2018.
24. Berry DA, Cronin KA, Plevritis SK, et al. Effect of screening and adjuvant therapy on mortality from breast cancer. N Engl J Med 2005;353(17):1784–92.
25. Iqbal J, Ginsburg O, Rochon PA, et al. Differences in breast cancer stage at diagnosis and cancer-specific survival by race and ethnicity in the United States. JAMA 2015;313(2):165–73.
26. Newman L. Breast cancer in African-American women. Oncologist 2005;10(1):1–14.
27. American Cancer Society. Cancer facts & figures for African Americans 2016-2018. Atlanta (GA): American Cancer Society; 2016.
28. Thomas DB, Gao DL, Ray RM, et al. Randomized trial of breast self-examination in Shanghai: final results. J Natl Cancer Inst 2002;94(19):1445–57.
29. Semiglazov VF, Sagaidak VN, Moiseyenko VM, et al. Study of the role of breast self-examination in the reduction of mortality from breast cancer. The Russian Federation/World Health Organization Study. Eur J Cancer 1993;29A(14):2039–46.

30. Mark K, Temkin SM, Terplan M. Breast self-awareness: the evidence behind the euphemism. Obstet Gynecol 2014;123(4):734–6.
31. Meissner HI, Klabunde CN, Han PK, et al. Breast cancer screening beliefs, recommendations and practices. Cancer 2011;117:3101–11.
32. McDonald S, Saslow D, Alciati MH. Performance and reporting of clinical breast examination: a review of the literature. CA Cancer J Clin 2004;54:345–61.
33. Fenton JJ, Barton MB, Geiger AM, et al. Screening clinical breast examination: how often does it miss lethal breast cancer? Natl Cancer Inst Monogr 2005;35:67–71.
34. Thistlethwaite J, Stewart RA. Clinical breast examination for asymptomatic women - exploring the evidence. Aust Fam Physician 2007;36(3):145–50.
35. Fenton JJ, Rolnick SJ, Harris EL, et al. Specificity of clinical breast examination in community practice. J Gen Intern Med 2007;22(3):332–7.
36. Ma I, Dueck A, Gray R, et al. Clinical and self breast examination remain important in the era of modern screening. Ann Surg Oncol 2012;19(5):1484–90.
37. Mouchawar J, Taplin S, Ichikawa L, et al. Late-stage breast cancer among women with recent negative screening mammography: do clinical encounters offer opportunity for earlier detection? J Natl Cancer Inst Monogr 2005;35:39–46.
38. Provencher L, Hogue JC, Desbiens C, et al. Is clinical breast examination important for breast cancer detection? Curr Oncol 2016;23(4):e332–9.
39. Pisani P, Parkin DM, Ngelangel C, et al. Outcome of screening by clinical examination of the breast in a trial in the Philippines. Int J Cancer 2006;118:149–54.
40. Boulos S, Gadallah M, Neguib S, et al. Breast screening in the emerging world: high prevalence of breast cancer in Cairo. Breast 2005;14:340–6.
41. Sankaranarayanan R, Ramadas K, Thara S, et al. Clinical breast examination: preliminary results from a cluster randomized controlled trial in India. J Natl Cancer Inst 2011;103(19):1476–80.
42. Miller AB, To T, Baines CJ, et al. Canadian National Breast Screening Study-2: 13-year results of a randomized trial in women aged 50-59 years. J Natl Cancer Inst 2000;92(18):1490–9.
43. Albert US, Schulz KD. Clinical breast examination: what can be recommended for its use to detect breast cancer in countries with limited resources? Breast J 2003;9(Suppl 2):S90–3.
44. Nelson HD, Cantor A, Humphrey L, et al. Screening for breast cancer: a systematic review to update the 2009 U.S. Preventive Services Task Force Recommendation. Evidence synthesis No. 124. AHRQ Publication No. 14-05201-EF-1. Rockville (MD): Agency for Healthcare Research and Quality; 2016.
45. Evidence summary: screening for breast cancer: breast cancer: screening. U.S. Preventive Services Task Force. 2016. Available at: https://www.uspreventiveservicestaskforce.org/Page/Document/RecommendationStatementFinal/breast-cancer-screening1. Accessed July 3, 2018.
46. Coldman AJ, Phillips N, Olivotto IA, et al. Impact of changing from annual to biennial mammographic screening on breast cancer outcomes in women aged 50-79 in British Columbia. J Med Screen 2008;15(4):182–7.
47. Parvinen I, Chiu S, Pylkkanen L, et al. Effects of annual vs triennial mammography interval on breast cancer incidence and mortality in ages 40-49 in Finland. Br J Cancer 2011;105(9):1388–91.
48. Available at: https://www.aafp.org/patient-care/clinical-recommendations/all/breast-cancer.html. Accessed July 2, 2018.

49. Oeffinger KC, Fontham ET, Etzioni R, et al. Breast cancer screening for women at average risk 2015 guideline update from the American Cancer Society. JAMA 2015;314(15):1599–614.
50. Committee on Practice Bulletins—Gynecology. Practice bulletin number 179: breast cancer risk assessment and screening in average-risk women. American College of Obstetricians and Gynecologists. Obstet Gynecol 2017;130:e1–16.
51. Monticciolo DL, Newell MS, Hendrick RE, et al. Breast cancer screening for average-risk women: recommendations from the ACR Commission on breast imaging. J Am Coll Radiol 2017;14(9):1137–43.
52. Monticciolo DL, Newell MS, Moy L, et al. Breast cancer screening in women at higher-than-average risk: recommendations from the ACR. J Am Coll Radiol 2018;15(3):408–14.
53. Ebell MH, Thai TN, Royalty KJ. Cancer screening recommendations: an international comparison of high income countries. Public Health Rev 2018;39(1):1.
54. Broeders M, Moss S, Nyström L, et al. The impact of mammography screening on breast cancer mortality in Europe: a review of observational studies. J Med Screen 2012;19:14–25.
55. Gorini G, Zappa M, Miccinesi G, et al. Breast cancer mortality trends in two areas of the province of Florence, Italy, where screening programmes started in the 1970s and 1990s. Br J Cancer 2004;90(9):1780–3.
56. Ascunce EN, Moreno-Iribas C, Barcos Urtiaga A, et al. Changes in breast cancer mortality in Navarre (Spain) after introduction of a screening programme. J Med Screen 2007;14(1):14–20.
57. Duffy SW, Tabár L, Olsen AH, et al. Absolute numbers of lives saved and over-diagnosis in breast cancer screening, from a randomized trial and from the Breast Screening Programme in England. J Med Screen 2010;17(1):25–30.
58. Hubbard RA, Kerlikowske K, Flowers CI, et al. Cumulative probability of false-positive recall or biopsy recommendation after 10 years of screening mammography: a cohort study. Ann Intern Med 2011;155(8):481–92.
59. Available at: https://www.Breastcancer.org. Accessed July 2, 2018.
60. Committee opinion no. 625: management of women with dense breasts diagnosed by mammography. American College of Obstetricians and Gynecologists. Obstet Gynecol 2015;125:750–1.
61. Evidence summary: supplemental screening in women with dense breasts: breast cancer: screening. U.S. Preventive Services Task Force. 2016. Available at: https://www.uspreventiveservicestaskforce.org/Page/Document/evidence-summary-supplemental-screening-in-women-with-dense-/breast-cancer-screening1. Accessed July 19, 2018.
62. Lee CH, Dershaw DD, Kopans D, et al. Breast cancer screening with imaging: recommendations from the Society of Breast Imaging and the ACR on the use of mammography, breast MRI, breast ultrasound, and other technologies for the detection of clinically occult breast cancer. J Am Coll Radiol 2010;7(1):18–27.
63. Gartlehner G, Thaler KJ, Chapman A, et al. Adjunct ultrasonography for breast cancer screening in women at average risk: a systematic review. Int J Evid Based Healthc 2013;11(2):87–93.
64. American Cancer Insitute. Available at: https://www.cancer.org/cancer/breast-cancer/screening-tests-and-early-detection/breast-mri-scans.html. Accessed July 1, 2018.
65. USPSTF published final recommendations. Available at: https://www.uspreventiveservicestaskforce.org/Page/Document/UpdateSummaryFinal/breast-cancer-screening1. Accessed July 2, 2018.

66. Moon HJ, Kim EK. Characteristics of breast cancer detected by supplementary screening ultrasonography. Ultrasonography 2015;34(3):153–6.
67. Paluch-Shimon S, Cardoso F, Sessa C, et al. Prevention and screening in BRCA mutation carriers and other breast/ovarian hereditary cancer syndromes: ESMO clinical practice guidelines for cancer prevention and screening. Ann Oncol 2016;27(suppl_5):v103–10.
68. Oshima Lee E, Emanuel EJ. Shared decision making to improve care and reduce costs. N Engl J Med 2013;368(1):6–8.

Cervical Cancer and Its Precursors

A Preventative Approach to Screening, Diagnosis, and Management

Sarah E. Stumbar, MD, MPH[a],*, Maria Stevens, MD[a], Zoe Feld, MD[b]

KEYWORDS

- Cervical cancer • Human papillomavirus vaccine • Papanicolaou test
- Cervical intraepithelial neoplasia • Colposcopy

KEY POINTS

- Screening for cervical cancer—through cytology testing, human papilloma virus testing, or a combination of the two—looks to detect preinvasive disease, thereby allowing for medical intervention before invasive disease has developed.
- Although human papilloma virus DNA is present in the majority of cervical cancers, there are a myriad other risk factors that impact a woman's likelihood of developing the disease.
- Cervical cancer screening has resulted in declines in disease incidence and mortality, with the majority of new cervical cancer cases occurring in women who have never or rarely been screened.
- Guidelines surrounding the type of screening, optimal interval, and risk–benefit considerations continue to evolve as new data emerges.
- Vaccination against high-risk human papillomavirus is the most direct targeted strategy for cervical cancer prevention.

CLINICAL DESCRIPTION OF DISEASE

Cervical cancer affects the cells lining the cervix, most commonly occurring in the cells of the transformation zone, which is the part of the cervix where the glandular cells of the endocervix meet the squamous cells of the exocervix. Approximately 70% of cervical cancers are of the squamous cell type and nearly 25% are of the adenocarcinoma type that develop from glandular cells. Other types of cervical cancer may

Disclosure: The authors have nothing to disclose.
[a] Department of Humanities, Health, and Society, Herbert Wertheim College of Medicine, Florida International University, 11200 Southwest 8th Street, Miami, FL 33199, USA;
[b] Department of Obstetrics and Gynecology, University of California, Davis, Davis, CA, USA
* Corresponding author. 11200 Southwest 8th Street, AHC2-584, Miami, FL 33199.
E-mail address: sstumbar@fiu.edu

also occur, but are extremely rare.[1] Cervical cancer generally develops over the course of many years; precancerous changes—called cervical intraepithelial neoplasia (CIN), dysplasia, or squamous intraepithelial neoplasia—evolve first, and then slowly progress from precancer to cancer over a period of 10 to 20 years.[2,3]

Importantly, screening for cervical cancer—either with cytology through the Papanicolaou test (Pap smear), human papillomavirus (HPV) testing, or a combination of the two—looks to detect preinvasive disease, thereby allowing for medical intervention before invasive disease has developed.[4] Cervical cancer precursors include cytologic findings of atypical squamous cells of undetermined significance and low-grade squamous intraepithelial lesions (LSIL) and histologic findings of mild dysplasia, called CIN1. Precancerous cervical lesions include cytologic findings of high-grade squamous intraepithelial lesions and atypical glandular cells and histologic findings of more advanced dysplasia, called CIN2 and CIN3.[2] CIN lesions result from a complex interaction between high-risk HPV types and immature metaplastic cervical epithelium.[5]

Pathogenesis and Risk Factors

HPV is the most common sexually transmitted disease in the United States among both men and women, with about 14 million cases diagnosed annually.[6] HPV is associated with a myriad of cancers, including those of the cervix, oropharynx, penis, and anus. Most cervical HPV infections are transient and are cleared from the body within 6 to 24 months.[7] However, nearly all cervical cancers are associated with persistent infection by high-risk HPV types, including 16, 18, 31, 33, 45, 52, and 58.[8] Specifically, HPV types 16 and 18 are found in more than 70% of cervical cancers.[9] Most women with HPV infection do not develop CIN or cervical cancer and, even when the natural course of the disease is not altered by biopsy or other medical intervention, fewer than one-third of low-grade CIN will progress to high-grade lesions and the majority of high grade CIN does not advance to invasive cervical cancer.[6]

The factors that determine persistence of HPV infection or progression of disease are not fully understood. In an immunocompetent host, it seems that HPV infection alone is not sufficient for a woman to develop invasive cervical cancer; rather, she needs to be exposed to other cervical cancer risk factors or carcinogenic events over many years before cervical cancer develops.[6,10] Although HPV DNA is present in the majority of cervical cancers, there are a myriad other risk factors that impact a woman's likelihood of developing the disease. These risk factors are included in **Table 1**.

Intrauterine devices (IUDs) have been shown to be protective against progression to invasive cervical cancer. This protective effect may be explained by a local cellular immune response induced by the IUD, which helps the body to clear itself of the HPV infection. The protective effect of an IUD starts after less than 1 year of use and persists after the IUD has been removed.[13,19]

Symptoms

Early stage cervical cancers are generally asymptomatic, thereby emphasizing the importance of routine screening. If symptoms do occur, irregular or heavy vaginal bleeding and postcoital bleeding are most common. A nonspecific vaginal discharge may also occur. Advanced cervical cancer may present with nonspecific pelvic or lower back pain; a myriad bowel or bladder symptoms, including pelvic pressure, hematuria, hematochezia, or vaginal passage of urine or stool indicating fistula formation, may also occur in advanced disease, but are uncommon.[20]

Table 1 Cervical cancer risk factors	
Risk Factor	**Comments**
Human papillomavirus infection	Human papillomavirus DNA is present in 99% of cervical cancers[11]; infection is thought to be necessary but not sufficient to develop cervical cancer.
Immunocompromised state	Immunocompromised women are at increased risk of developing invasive cervical cancer; this includes women on chronic immunosuppressive therapy, such as steroids, and women with human immunodeficiency virus.[12]
Smoking	Women who smoke are about twice as likely to develop cervical cancer as those who do not smoke.[13] Cotinine, nicotine, and other tobacco byproducts have been detected in cervical mucosa, and may impair the local immune response and damage cervical epithelial cells, thereby increasing the risk of developing progressive disease.[14,15]
Oral contraceptive pills	The risk of cervical cancer increases proportionally to the duration of oral contraceptive pill use and decreases after cessation of use.[16]
Multiple pregnancies	Women with ≥5 pregnancies were nearly twice as likely as women with 1–2 pregnancies to develop cervical cancer.[17] It is unclear why this association exists. Hormonal changes during pregnancy may make women more susceptible to HPV infection and cancer growth, or a weakened immune system during pregnancy may allow cervical cancer to develop.[12]
Exposure to diethylstilbestrol	Diethylstilbestrol was used to prevent pregnancy complications before 1971; it has been shown to be associated with a myriad negative health outcomes, including increased risk for cervical intraepithelial neoplasia grade ≥2.[18]
Lower socioeconomic status	Women of lower socioeconomic statuses are less likely to get regular Pap smear testing, and thereby are less likely to get diagnosed with and treated for preinvasive cervical disease. This increases their risk of eventually being diagnosed with invasive cervical cancer.
Age at first parity	In Studies, Women who experienced parity before age 17 had nearly 3 times the risk of developing cervical cancer than those who experienced parity after age 25.[17]
Number of sex partner	In Studies, Women with ≥6 sex partners were about 3 times as likely to develop cervical cancer as those with one sex partner.[17]

Course of the Disease and Staging

Invasive cervical cancers can spread by the lymphatic system, hematogenously, or via direct extension. Direct extension most commonly invades the uterine corpus, vagina, parametria, peritoneal cavity, bladder, or rectum; the ovaries are rarely effected.[21] The lungs, liver, and bone are the most common sites of hematogenous spread. Studies have shown that any pelvic lymph node group may be impacted.[22]

The International Federation of Gynecology and Obstetrics 2014 guideline is most often used for staging cervical cancer.[23] Unlike other gynecologic cancers, cervical cancer is staged clinically before surgery, and staging is based on tumor size and depth of invasion, direct spread into surrounding tissues, and distant metastases. A combination of MRI, computed tomography scans, and PET scans is used to assist in the evaluation of both the primary tumor and metastatic disease.[24] **Table 2**

Table 2	
International Federation of Gynecology and Obstetrics (FIGO) staging for cervical cancer	
FIGO Stage	**Stage Description**
I	Cancer has not spread beyond the cervix. Extension to the uterine corpus is not considered.
IA	Invasive cancer can only be seen with assistance of microscope. Invasion of stroma is $\leq$5 mm deep and $\leq$7 mm wide.
IA1	Invasion of stroma is $\leq$3 mm deep and $\leq$7 mm wide.
IA2	Invasion of stroma is between 3 and 5 mm deep and <7 mm wide.
IB	Stage I cancers that can be seen without a microscope or can only be seen with a microscope and are deeper than 5 mm or wider than 7 mm.
IB1	Cancer can be seen without a microscope and is <4 cm.
IB2	Cancer can be seen without a microscope and is larger than 4 cm.
II	Cancer has grown beyond the cervix and uterus, but hasn't invaded the walls of the pelvis or lower one-third of the vagina.
IIA	Cancer has not spread into the parametria.
IIA1	Cancer can be seen without a microscope but is <4 cm.
IIA2	Cancer can be seen without a microscope and is >4 cm.
IIB	Cancer has spread into the parametria.
III	Cancer has spread to the walls of the pelvis or lower one-third of the vagina or is causing hydronephrosis.
IIIA	Cancer has spread to the lower one-third of the vagina without extension to the walls of the pelvis.
IIIB	Cancer has spread to the walls of the pelvis and/or is causing hydronephrosis.
IV	Cancer has spread beyond the pelvis or has involved the mucosa of the bladder or rectum.
IVA	Cancer has spread to adjacent organs
IVB	Cancer has spread to distant organs

Data from FIGO Committee on Gynecologic Oncology. FIGO staging for carcinoma of the vulva, cervix, and corpus uteri. Int J Gynaecol Obstet 2014;125(2):97–8.

describes the International Federation of Gynecology and Obstetrics stages for cervical cancer; these range from stage I (least advanced disease) to stage IV (most advanced disease).

Treatment

The treatment of cervical cancer is guided by cancer stage, and by the patient's comorbidities, risk for recurrence, and fertility goals.[24] Treatment options include surgical intervention, chemotherapy, radiation therapy, or a combination. Depending on the stage of cancer and fertility goals of the patient, surgical intervention may include cone biopsy, tachelectomy (removal of the cervix and parts of the vagina), or hysterectomy.[25] The type of hysterectomy depends on disease stage and may be performed using a laparoscopic or robotic approach. Microinvasive cervical cancers may be treated with simple hysterectomy, whereas more advanced disease requires radical hysterectomy, which removes lymph tissue and, to a variable extent, portions of the vagina, parametria, and bladder.[24] Depending on disease invasion and spread, chemotherapy and radiation may also be part of the treatment regimen; stage IV cervical cancer is generally considered not to be curable, and chemotherapy and radiation are used to slow disease progression and palliate the patient's symptoms.[26]

Treatment of disease recurrence depends on the patient's previous treatments and the extent of recurrent disease. In localized recurrence, hysterectomy is again an option, and may include exenteration, a surgical procedure that removes the female reproductive organs, lower urinary tract, and part of the rectosigmoid. Although exenteration has a 50% cure rate, it also carries a 3% to 5% mortality rate and one-half of patients experience major complications.[26,27]

EPIDEMIOLOGY
Screening Rates

Cervical cancer screening has resulted in well-documented declines in incidence and mortality in the United States.[28] Most new cervical cancer cases occur in women who have never or rarely been screened.[29] For example, the Southern United States experiences a higher cervical cancer disease burden while also reporting lower HPV vaccine uptake and Pap smear screening rates.[30]

As such, Healthy People 2020 includes goals to increase screening rates for breast, cervical, and colorectal cancers. For cervical cancer, the goal is a 93% screening rate.[31] A 2017 study used data from the National Health Interview Survey to look at national cancer screening rates, along with a number of factors associated with screening disparities.[32] This analysis found that, in 2015, 83% of women reported being up to date with cervical cancer screening, with no evident increase in this rate between 2000 and 2015; this falls well short of the Healthy People 2020 cervical cancer screening goal. Furthermore, there were persistent disparities in screening rates based on race/ethnicity, socioeconomic status, and other health care access indicators. Among uninsured women, the reported cervical cancer screening rate was only 63.9%; whereas 86.3% of privately insured women reported being up to date with cervical cancer screening. Women without a regular health care source reported screening rates of 65.1%; this rate increased to 85.5% for women with a regular source of health care. There were also distinct racial/ethnic differences in screening rates; Asian women reported the lowest rates of screening, at 75.8%. Seventy-nine percent of Hispanic women, compared with 83.7% of non-Hispanic women, reported being up to date with screening. The proportion of women reporting up-to-date cervical cancer screening increased proportionally and significantly with educational level and income.[28]

Incidence and Outcomes

The National Cancer Institute estimates that 12,820 women were diagnosed with cervical cancer in 2017, representing 0.8% of all cancer diagnoses. In the same year, 4210 women died of cervical cancer, representing 0.7% of all deaths from cancer. From 2007 to 2013, 47% of women were diagnosed with localized disease, 36% were diagnosed with regional disease, and 14% with distant metastatic disease.[33,34] The 5-year survival rates based on cervical cancer stage at diagnosis can be found in **Table 3**.

From 1983 through 2009, there were definite improvements in 5-year survival rates for women who were diagnosed with localized, early stage cervical cancer, but little improvement was seen for women diagnosed with distant disease.[35] It is important to note that there are well-documented, persistent racial and geographic disparities in 5-year survival rates, with white women experiencing more favorable outcomes.[34,36]

SCREENING RECOMMENDATIONS

Guidelines surrounding the type of screening, optimal interval, and risk–benefit considerations continue to evolve as new data emerges. There are currently 3 main

Table 3	
Cervical cancer stage at diagnosis and reported 5-year survival rates	
Cervical Cancer AJCC Stage at Diagnosis	5-Year Survival Rate (%)
Stage IA	93
Stage IB	80
Stage IIA	63
Stage IIB	58
Stage IIIA	35
Stage IIIB	32
Stage IVA	16
Stage IVB	15

Data from AJCC cancer staging manual. 7th edition. New York: Springer; 2010.

options for screening: cytology, HPV testing, and visual inspection (**Fig. 1**). Selection depends on the age of the patient and type of resources available in the population being screened. In the United States, the wide use of both cytology and HPV testing is standard of care. However, in developing countries and very low resource settings, visual inspection can serve as a safe and effective alternative.[37] It is important to note that all screening methods offer substantial benefit in terms of reducing cancer incidence and mortality; thus, any screening is better than no screening.

Conventional Versus Liquid-Based Pap Smear

The first cytology test developed required cervical specimens to be collected and placed directly onto a glass slide for microscopic interpretation. Although this conventional method proved to be effective in detecting cervical cancer, a more practical technology known as the liquid based pap was later developed. In the liquid based preparation, the sample is deposited in a small bottle of preservative fluid and sent to the laboratory. This test is more widely used owing to its convenience, reduction in laboratory time, and improvement in rate of inadequate samples. However, both are acceptable screening tools in terms of their efficacy.[38]

Human Papillomavirus Testing

Testing for HPV is standard of care across most practices (**Fig. 2**). It was initially used as a reflex test to risk stratify women aged 21 years and older with a cytology

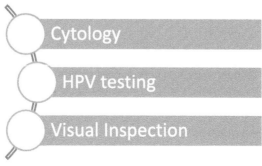

Fig. 1. Methods available for cervical cancer screening. HPV, human papillomavirus.

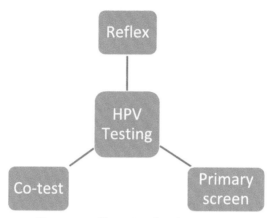

Fig. 2. Options for use of human papillomavirus (HPV) testing in cervical cancer screening.

diagnosis of atypical squamous cells of undetermined significance and postmeno-pausal women with a cytology diagnosis of LSIL.[39] Then it became implemented as an adjunct to cytology or a co-test in women older than 30 years to lengthen the rec-ommended interval time for screening. Now the latest change has emerged with the US Food and Drug Administration approval of the first high-risk HPV test made spe-cifically for primary cervical cancer screening. Data from several large randomized controlled trials show primary screening to be equivalent or superior to current cytology based methods.[40] Many of the leading medical organizations have updated, or are in the processing of updating, their existing guidelines and recommendations to support its use.

Age-Based Recommendations

Choosing the appropriate time frame and interval for screening is important to maximize benefit and minimize harm to patients. As our knowledge of HPV and methods for testing evolve, there have been several changes to the recom-mended age and time intervals of screening. **Fig. 3** summarizes recommendations from the US Preventive Services Task Force,[41] American Congress of Obstetri-cians and Gynecologists,[42] American Cancer Society,[42] American Society for Col-poscopy and Cervical Pathology (ASCCP),[40] and the Society of Gynecologic Oncology.[40] These are screening guidelines and therefore apply to asymptomatic women only. They do not apply to women who have been diagnosed with a high-grade precancerous cervical lesion, cervical cancer, women with in utero exposure to diethylstilbestrol, or immunocompromised individuals who are at high risk for cervical cancer, such as women living with human immunodeficiency virus infection.

- In women younger than 21 years of age, transient cervical dysplasia is common and the incidence of cervical cancer is extremely low. Thus, regardless of the age of onset of sexual activity, screening in this age group should be avoided because it can lead to unnecessary testing and harm.
- The consensus among all guidelines is to start screening at 21 years of age. Testing with cytology alone every 3 years between the ages of 21 and 29 was previously the sole method of testing for this age group, and the US Pre-ventive Services Task Force continues to support this recommendation.

Less than 21

- No screening recommended (ASCCP, ACS, USPSTF, ACOG)

21 to 29

- Cytology alone every 3 y (ASCCP, ACS, USPSTF, ACOG)
    - OR
- High-risk HPV testing alone every 3 y for women *25 and older* (ASCCP, SGO)

30 to 65

- Cytology alone every 3 y (USPSTF, ACOG)
    OR
- High-risk HPV testing alone every 3 y (ASCCP, SGO) or every 5 y (USPSTF).
    OR
- Cotesting every 5 y (USPSTF, ACOG)

65 and older

- No screening recommended if adequate history of negative screening results and not at high risk for cervical cancer (ASCCP, ACS, USPSTF, ACOG)

Fig. 3. Age-based screening guidelines for cervical cancer, including the use of cytology and human papillomavirus (HPV) testing. ACOG, American Congress of Obstetricians and Gynecologists; ACS, American Cancer Society; ASCCP, American Society for Colposcopy and Cervical Pathology; SGO, Society of Gynecologic Oncology; USPSTF, US Preventive Services Task Force. (*Data from* Refs.[39,42,43])

However, interim guidance released by the ASCCP and Society of Gynecologic Oncology supports primary HPV screening in women age 25 years or older as an alternative to current cytology-based screening.

- For women ages 30 to 65, cytology with high-risk HPV cotesting is currently the consensus guideline among all organizations. However, the US Preventive Services Task Force is currently considering high-risk HPV screening alone as an alternative to cytology." with "For women ages 30 to 65, multiple screening strategies exist, including Pap smear testing alone, high risk HPV testing alone, and co-testing. The recommended screening interval is either every 3 or 5 years, depending on the chosen modality. There is no evidence clearly indicating that one method is superior to another.[41]
- Based on theoretic modeling, studies show it is reasonable to discontinue cervical cancer screening at 65 years of age. This decision should be made only after determining if the patient has received adequate screening and is at low risk. Adequate screening is defined as 3 consecutive negative cytology results or 2 negative results in a row within the past 10 years, with the most recent test performed within the last 5 years.
- Screening should be discontinued in women who have had a hysterectomy with removal of the cervix for benign indications. Women with a history of cancer or high-grade cervical intraepithelial lesions before hysterectomy are at risk and should continue to be screened.[1]

Overall, there are no data or guidelines that support routine annual screening. Screening more frequently than every 3 years can lead to procedures with unwanted adverse effects such as cervical incompetence and preterm labor.[43] Adopting a 5-year screening interval strategy may offer the best balance of benefits and harms. It is important to clearly explain and communicate new recommendations to patients to gain their acceptance and adherence with screening. The greatest focus should be placed on receiving regular adequate screening, regardless of the method or interval used.

PREVENTION RECOMMENDATIONS

Although cervical cancer prevention strategies can include behavioral interventions directed toward limiting number of sexual partners, condom use, and reduction in cigarette smoking, vaccination against high-risk HPV represents the most direct targeted strategy.[44]

There are 3 HPV vaccines approved by the US Food and Drug Administration for use in the United States, although only the 9-valent GARDASIL vaccine is currently in use.[45] All 3 are L1 protein vaccines that induce the formation of neutralizing antibodies against HPV 6, 11, 16, and 18, and some other HPV genotypes. With the availability of the HPV vaccine since 2007, the prevalence of high-risk HPV infection has decreased by up to 64% in the target population of adolescent women for whom the vaccine had been recommended.[46] Furthermore, all 3 vaccines have been shown to decrease the risk of CIN 1, CIN 2, and CIN 3 by more than 95%.[47] **Table 4** contains more details about each of the HPV vaccines that are currently available in the United States.

The Centers for Disease Control and Prevention's Advisory Committee on Immunization Practices recommends routine HPV vaccination for both sexes starting at age 11 or 12 years, and as early as age 9 years. Recent changes in guidelines indicate that females and males who were not adequately vaccinated previously may receive the vaccine until age 45. For individuals who initiate the vaccine after the age of 15 years, as well as for those with primary or secondary immune compromise, a 3-dose vaccine schedule is recommended, with the second dose administered 1 to 2 months after the first and the third dose administered 6 months after the first dose.[41] For children under age 15 years, a 2-dose schedule is now recommended, with the administration of the second dose 6 to 12 months after the first dose. The implementation of a 2-dose schedule increases convenience for providers, parents, and vaccine recipients. With a decrease in costs, resources, and logistical challenges, the 2-dose schedule is expected to result in an increased proportion of children under age 15 who have completed the recommended series.[41,48,49]

It is important to note that vaccination will not entirely eliminate the need for cervical cancer screening in the United States because not all HPV types that cause cervical cancer are included in the vaccines currently in use.[50] Therefore, vaccination is not a substitute for routine cervical cancer screening and vaccinated patients should undergo cervical cancer screening as recommended. However, there is ongoing research examining whether guidelines should be modified based on a woman's vaccination status.[51]

The HPV vaccine has rarely been associated with anaphylactic and hypersensitivity reactions. The most common adverse reactions to the vaccine include[52]:

- Injection site reaction,
- Headache,
- Fever,
- Nausea,
- Dizziness,
- Diarrhea,
- Pharyngolaryngeal pain,
- Vomiting,
- Cough, and
- Fatigue.

Table 4
Currently available vaccines against human papilloma virus (HPV)

Vaccine	Manufacturer/ Year of License	Genotypes	Availability/Cost	Schedule/Administration	Efficacy	Considerations
GARDASIL 9 (9vHPV)	Merck and Co., 2014	6, 11, 16, 18 31, 33, 45, 52, 58	Out-of-pocket expense: $214.99–$249.99 per dose[11,12]	Two-dose schedule for males and females under age 15, with second dose 6–12 mo after first Three-dose schedule for those >15 y with second dose 1–2 mo after, and third dose 6 mo after first[41]	97.4% for prevention of high-grade cervical, vulvar and vaginal disease related to HPV 31, 33, 45, 52, and 58[14] Demonstrated noninferiority in efficacy compared with Cervarix[15]	The only high-risk HPV vaccine currently in use in the United States; covers Gardasil strains and 5 additional high-risk oncogenic strains that account for 15% of cervical cancers[16]
GARDASIL (4vHPV)	Merck and Co., 2007	6, 11, 16, 18	Not in use in the United States, as of 2016[41]	3 doses: 0, 1, and 6 mo	93%–100% for prevention of cytologic abnormalities associated with HPV types 6, 11, 16 or 18[17,18,h]	HPV types 16 and 18 associated with 70% of cervical cancers; HPV types 6 and 11 cause 90% of genital warts
Cervarix (2vHPV)	GlaxoSmithKline, 2009	16, 18	Not in use in the United States, as of 2016[41]	3 doses: 0, 1, and 6 mo	91%–93% for prevention of cytologic abnormalities associated with HPV types 16 or 18[41]	Cervarix is the most cost-effective vaccine with proven efficacy in 1 dose and has demonstrated sustained high antibody titers for ≥10 y[46]

Table 5
Potential outcomes of cervical cancer screening, including human papillomavirus (HPV) and cytology results

Outcomes of Cervical Cancer Screening	Comments
HR HPV 16 HR HPV 18	High-risk carcinogenic serotype; together account for 25% of low-grade lesions, 50%–60% of high-grade lesions, and 70% of invasive cervical cancers
HR HPV other	May include genotypes 31, 45, 10, 26, 33, 35, 39, 51, 52, 55, 56, 58, 59, 66, 68
LSIL	Low-grade squamous intraepithelial lesion
HSIL	High-grade squamous intraepithelial lesion
ASC-US	Atypical cells of undetermined significance; ASC-US is the most common abnormal Pap test result
ASC-H	Atypical squamous cells, concern for the presence of HSIL
AGC	Atypical glandular cells
AIS	Adenocarcinoma in situ

Abbreviations: AGC, atypical glandular cells; AIS, adenocarcinoma in situ; ASC-US, atypical squamous cells of undetermined significance; HR, high risk; HSIL, high-grade squamous intraepithelial lesion; LSIL, low-grade squamous intraepithelial lesion.
Data from Gordon J. Obstetrics, gynecology & infertility. Arlington (VA): Scrub Hill Press; 2016.

The GARDASIL 9 vaccine is an US Food and Drug Administration pregnancy category B medication and, although no adverse fetal effects of vaccination during pregnancy have been found, it is not recommended for use during pregnancy. It is unknown whether vaccine antigens or antibodies induced by HPV vaccines are excreted in breast milk, but breastfeeding is not a contraindication to receiving the HPV vaccine.[53]

OUTCOMES AND COMPLICATIONS OF CERVICAL CANCER SCREENING

Potential outcomes of cervical cancer screening include normal and abnormal screening results. Normal results may include negative cytology and/or the absence of HPV depending on the testing strategy used and, in these instances, the resumption of screening at the recommended, routine intervals is indicated (generally either every

Table 6
Possible abnormal results of colposcopic biopsy

Abnormal Outcomes of Colposcopy	Comments
CIN 1	CIN, mild dysplasia; dysplastic cells are confined to the deeper layers (lower third) of the epithelium
CIN 2	CIN, moderate dysplasia; dysplastic cellular changes restricted to the lower two-thirds of the epithelium, with more marked nuclear abnormalities than in CIN 1
CIN 3	CIN, severe dysplasia; nuclear abnormalities extend throughout the thickness of the epithelium
CS	Carcinoma in situ

Abbreviation: CIN, cervical intraepithelial neoplasia.

Table 7
Cumulative risks of persistent human papillomavirus (HPV) infection, cervical intraepithelial neoplasia (CIN)2, CIN3, and cancer among 32,374 women aged 30 to 64 years testing HPV-positive/Pap-negative at baseline

Baseline Screening Results		Follow-up Results At 1 Year				Follow-up Results at 2 Years				Follow-up Results at 5 Years			
Cytology	HPV status	HPV status	CIN2	CIN3	Cancer	HPV status	CIN2	CIN3	Cancer	HPV status	CIN2	CIN3	Cancer
Negative	Positive	56% HPV positive	2.8%	1.1%	0.11%	37% HPV positive	4.8%	2.0%	0.17%	12% HPV positive	10%	4.5%	0.34%

Data from Katki H, Schiffman M, Castle P, et al. Five-year risks of CIN 3+ and cervical cancer among women who test Pap-negative but are HPV-positive. J Low Genit Tract Dis 2013;17:S56–63.

3 or every 5 years). Abnormal results may include various pathologic cytology findings or the presence of certain HPV genotypes. **Table 5** lists potential outcomes of cervical cancer screening, including HPV and cytology results.[45]

The ASCCP collaborated with 23 other national organizations to produce the Updated Consensus Guidelines for Managing Abnormal Cervical Cancer Screening Tests, which were released in 2012. These guidelines provide algorithms for managing Pap smear testing results based on patient age, cervical cancer screening history, and current cytology and HPV result. These clinically useful algorithms can be accessed via the ASCCP website or mobile app.

In accordance with ASCCP recommendations, abnormal Pap smear screening test results may be followed up with colposcopy.[2] Colposcopy is a diagnostic procedure used to identify precancerous and cancerous lesions. Colposcopic visualization is indicated for the following Pap smear findings[2]:

- Persistent atypical squamous cells of undetermined significance or AS-US with high-risk HPV positive,
- Normal cytology but persistent high-risk HPV positive,
- ASC-H,
- Atypical glandular cells,
- Low-grade squamous intraepithelial lesion with unknown HPV or high-risk HPV positive for those greater than 30 years of age,
- Low-grade squamous intraepithelial lesion in those 25 to 29 years of age,
- High-grade squamous intraepithelial lesions, and
- Malignant cells.

Colposcopy involves the examination of the cervix, vagina, and vulva using a colposcope after application of 3% to 5% acetic acid solution. It is combined with obtaining colposcopically directed biopsies of all lesions that seem to be suspicious for neoplasia. A colposcopy is considered satisfactory if the entire squamocolumnar junction and the margin of any visible lesion can be seen with the colposcope. Satisfactory colposcopy can result in a normal result, with the absence of any dysplasia or neoplasia, or an abnormal result of CIN. Final diagnosis of CIN is established by the histopathologic examination of an excised specimen. CIN may be categorized into grades 1, 2, and 3 depending on the proportion of the thickness of the epithelium

Table 8
Cytology and human papillomavirus (HPV) status in women 30 to 64 years of age and associated cumulative 5-year risk of cervical intraepithelial neoplasia (CIN)2, CIN3, and invasive cervical cancer

Cytology	HPV Status	5-Year Risk of CIN2 (%)	5-Year Risk of CIN3 (%)	5-Year Risk of Cancer (%)
Negative	Negative	0.27	0.08	0.011
ASC-US	Negative	1.10	0.43	—
LSIL	Negative	5.10	2.00	—
Negative	Positive	10.00	4.50	0.340
ASC-US	Positive	18.00	6.80	0.410
LSIL	Positive	19.00	6.10	0.089

Abbreviations: ASC-US, atypical squamous cells of undetermined significance; LSIL, low-grade squamous intraepithelial lesion.

Data from Katki H, Schiffman M, Castle P, et al. Five-year risks of CIN 3+ and cervical cancer among women who test Pap-negative but are HPV-positive. J Low Genit Tract Dis 2013;17:S56–63.

Table 9
Potential adverse effects of colposcopy procedures

	Adverse Effect (%)		
Procedure	Pain	Bleeding	Discharge
Colposcopy examination only	14–18		
Colposcopy with biopsy	53	79	46
Colposcopy with large loop excision	67	87	63

Data from The TOMBOLA Trial of Management of Borderline and Other Low-grade Abnormal smears Group. After-effects reported by women following colposcopy, cervical biopsies and LLETZ: results from the TOMBOLA trial. BJOG 2009;116(11):1506–14.

showing mature and differentiated cells. The possible abnormal results of colposcopic biopsies are included in **Table 6**.[2]

Depending on the Pap smear cytology and HPV results, there is a variable risk of progression to CIN and invasive cervical cancer. These risks are outlined in **Tables 7** and **8**.

The diagnostic and therapeutic procedures related to cervical cancer screening carry risk for complications; the most common are pain, bleeding, discharge, and anxiety.[54] The risks of these complications is outlined in **Table 9**. Educating women about the potential after effects of these procedures can alleviate anxiety and provide reassurance, thus minimizing the harms of screening. In addition, obstetric complications can result from procedural excision of the cervix, including cervical stenosis and cervical incompetence leading to miscarriage and preterm labor.[17]

SUMMARY

Cervical cancer affects the cells lining the cervix, most commonly occurring in the cells of the transformation zone. Persistent infection with the HPV is implicated in the vast majority of cervical cancer cases; other risk factors include smoking, immunocompromise, increasing number of sexual partners, increasing number of pregnancies, and lower socioeconomic status.

Screening for cervical cancer—either through the cytology testing with the Pap smear, HPV testing, or a combination—looks to detect preinvasive disease, thereby allowing for medical intervention before invasive disease has developed. Selection of screening method depends on the age of the patient, her previous cervical cancer screening history and results, and the resources available.

Cervical cancer screening has resulted in well-documented decreases in incidence and mortality in the United States. However, persistent racial and socioeconomic disparities in screening and the resulting disease burden exist; screening rates still fall short of the target levels set forth by Healthy People 2020. Guidelines surrounding the type of screening, optimal interval, and risk–benefit considerations continue to evolve as new data emerge. Screening guidelines are slowly shifting to recommend HPV testing alone, rather than HPV testing in combination with Pap smears.

Although cervical cancer prevention strategies can include behavioral interventions directed toward limiting number of sexual partners, increasing condom use, and reducing cigarette smoking, vaccination against high-risk HPV represents the most targeted prevention strategy. Primary care physicians play an integral role in following guidelines for HPV vaccination for their adolescent and young adult patients, and for implementing comprehensive and evidence-based cervical cancer screening practices.

REFERENCES

1. Ries LAG, Melbert D, Krapcho M, et al. SEER cancer statistics review, 1975-2004. Bethesda (MD): National Cancer Institute; 2007.
2. ASCCP. Algorithms-updated consensus guidelines for managing abnormal cervical cancer screening tests and cancer precursors. Available at: http://www.asccp.org/asccp-guidelines. Accessed June 20, 2018.
3. Schiffman M, Kjaer SK. Chapter 2: natural history of anogenital human papillomavirus infection and neoplasia. J Natl Cancer Inst Monogr 2003;31:14–9.
4. Subramaniam A, Fauci JM, Schneider KE, et al. Invasive cervical cancer and screening: what are the rates of unscreened and underscreened women in the modern era? J Low Genit Tract Dis 2011;15(2):110–3.
5. Cox JT. Epidemiology of cervical intraepithelial neoplasia: the role of human papillomavirus. Baillieres Clin Obstet Gynaecol 1995;9(1):1–37.
6. Satterwhite C, Torrone E, Meites E, et al. Sexually transmitted infections among US women and men: prevalence and incidence estimates, 2008. Sex Transm Dis 2013;40:187–93.
7. Rodriguez AC, Schiffman M, Herrero R, et al. Rapid clearance of human papillomavirus and implications for clinical focus on persistent infections. J Natl Cancer Inst 2008;100(7):513–7.
8. International Agency for Research on Cancer (IARC). IARC monographs on the evaluation of carcinogenic risks to humans: human papillomaviruses, vol. 90. Lyon (France): IARC Press/World Health Organization; 2007.
9. Li N, Franceschi S, Howell-Jones R, et al. Human papillomavirus type distribution in 30,848 invasive cervical cancers worldwide: variation by geographical region, histological type and year of publication. Int J Cancer 2011;128(4):927–35.
10. Arends MJ, Buckley CH, Wells M. Aetiology, pathogenesis and pathology of cervical neoplasia. J Clin Pathol 1998;51:96–103.
11. Saraiya M, Unger ER, Thompson TD, et al. US assessment of HPV types in cancers: implications for current and 9-valent HPV vaccines. J Natl Cancer Inst 2015; 107:djv086.
12. American Cancer Society. What are the risk factors for cervical cancer? Available at: www.cancer.org/cancer/cervical-cancer/causes-risks-prevention/risk-factors. html. Accessed January 20, 2018.
13. Kataja V, Syrjänen S, Yliskoski M, et al. Risk factors associated with cervical human papillomavirus infections: a case-control study. Am J Epidemiol 1993;138: 735–45.
14. Sasson IM, Haley NJ, Wynder EL, et al. Cigarette smoking and neoplasia of the uterine cervix: smoke constituents in cervical mucus. N Engl J Med 1985;312: 315–6.
15. Roteli-Martines CM, Panetta K, Avancini Ferreira Alves V, et al. Cigarette smoking and high-risk HPV DNA as predisposing factors for high-grade cervical intraepithelial neoplasia (CIN) in young Brazilian women. Acta Obstet Gynecol Scand 1998;77:678–82.
16. International Collaboration of Epidemiological Studies of Cervical Cancer, Appleby P, Beral V, Berrington de González A, et al. Cervical cancer and hormonal contraceptives: collaborative reanalysis of individual data for 16,573 women with cervical cancer and 35,509 women without cervical cancer from 24 epidemiological studies. Lancet 2007;370:1609–21.
17. International Collaboration of Epidemiological Studies of Cervical Cancer. Comparison of risk factors for invasive squamous cell carcinoma and

adenocarcinoma of the cervix: collaborative reanalysis of individual data on 8,097 women with squamous cell carcinoma and 1,374 women with adenocarcinoma from 12 epidemiological studies. Int J Cancer 2007;120(11):2525.

18. Hoover RN, Hyet M, Pfeiffer RM, et al. Adverse health outcomes in women exposed in utero to diethylstilbestrol. N Engl J Med 2011;365(14):1304–14.

19. Castellsagué X, Díaz M, Vaccarella S, et al. Intrauterine device use, cervical infection with human papillomavirus, and risk of cervical cancer: a pooled analysis of 26 epidemiological studies. Lancet Oncol 2011;12:1023–31.

20. DiSaia PJ, Creasman WT. Invasive cervical cancer. In: Clinical gynecologic oncology. 7th edition. Philadelphia: Mosby Elsevier; 2007. p. 55.

21. Sutton GP, Bundy BN, Delgado G, et al. Ovarian metastases in stage IB carcinoma of the cervix: a Gynecologic Oncology Group study. Am J Obstet Gynecol 1992;166(1 Pt 1):50.

22. Bader AA, Winter R, Haas J, et al. Where to look for the sentinel lymph node in cervical cancer. Am J Obstet Gynecol 2007;197(6):678.e1.

23. FIGO Committee on Gynecologic Oncology. FIGO staging for carcinoma of the vulva, cervix, and corpus uteri. Int J Gynaecol Obstet 2014;125(2):97–8.

24. Wipperman J, Neil T, Williams T. Cervical cancer: evaluation and management. Am Fam Physician 2018;97(7):449–54.

25. American Cancer Society. Treatment options for cervical cancer, by stage. Available at: https://www.cancer.org/cancer/cervical-cancer/treating/by-stage.html. Accessed June 21, 2018.

26. Höckel M, Dornhöfer N. Pelvic exenteration for gynaecological tumours: achievements and unanswered questions. Lancet Oncol 2006;7(10):837–47.

27. Berek JS, Howe C, Lagasse LD, et al. Pelvic exenteration for recurrent gynecologic malignancy: survival and morbidity analysis of the 45-year experience at UCLA. Gynecol Oncol 2005;99(1):153–9.

28. Howlader N, Noone AM, Krapcho M, et al. SEER cancer statistics review, 1975-2012. Available at: http://seer.cancer.gov/csr/1975_2012. Accessed April 21, 2018.

29. Leyden WA, Manos MM, Geiger AM, et al. Cervical cancer in women with comprehensive health care access: attributable factors in the screening process. J Natl Cancer Inst 2005;97:675–83.

30. Jemal A, Simard EP, Dorell C, et al. Annual report to the nation on the status of cancer, 1975-2009, featuring the burden and trends in human papillomavirus (HPV)-associated cancers and HPV vaccination coverage levels. J Natl Cancer Inst 2013;105(3):175–201.

31. Healthy people 2020. Cancer: objectives: C-15: increase the proportion of women who receive a cervical cancer screening based on the most recent guidelines. Available at: https://www.healthypeople.gov/2020/topics-objectives/topic/cancer/objectives. Accessed June 20, 2018.

32. White A, Thompson TD, White MC, et al. Cancer screening test use-United States, 2015. MMWR Morb Mortal Wkly Rep 2015;66(8):201–6.

33. National Cancer Institute. Cancer stat facts: cervical cancer. Available at: https://seer.cancer.gov/statfacts/html/cervix.html. Accessed April 21, 2018.

34. Razzaghi H, Saraiya M, Thompson T, et al. Five-year relative survival for human papillomavirus-associated cancer sites. Cancer 2018;124(1):203–11.

35. Wright JD, Chen L, Tergas AI, et al. Population-level trends in relative survival for cervical cancer. Am J Obstet Gynecol 2015;213:670.e1-7.

36. Benard VB, Watson M, Saraiya M, et al. Cervical cancer survival in the United States by race and stage (2001-2009): findings from the CONCRD-2 study. Cancer 2017;123(Suppl 24):5119–37.
37. Chen C, Yang Z, Li Z, et al. Accuracy of several cervical screening strategies for early detection of cervical cancer: a meta-analysis. Int J Gynecol Cancer 2012; 22(6):908–21.
38. Siebers AG, Klinkhamer PJ, Grefte JM, et al. Comparison of liquid-based cytology with conventional cytology for detection of cervical cancer precursors: a randomized controlled trial. JAMA 2009;302(16):1757–64 [Erratum appears in JAMA 2009;302(21):2322].
39. American College of Obstetricians and Gynecologists. Cervical cytology screening. ACOG practice bulletin no. 109. Obstet Gynecol 2009;114:1409–20.
40. Huh WK, Ault KA, Chelmow D, et al. Use of primary high-risk human papillomavirus testing for cervical cancer screening: interim clinical guidance. Obstet Gynecol 2015;125(2):330–7.
41. U.S. Preventive Services Task Force. Cervical Cancer: Screening. 2018. Available at: https://www.uspreventiveservicestaskforce.org/Page/Document/UpdateSummaryFinal/cervical-cancer-screening2?ds=1&s=cervical%20cancer. Accessed November 21, 2018.
42. Saslow D, Solomon D, Lawson HW, et al. American Cancer Society, American Society for Colposcopy and Cervical Pathology, and American Society for Clinical Pathology screening guidelines for the prevention and early detection of cervical cancer. CA Cancer J Clin 2012;62:147–72.
43. U.S. Preventive Services Task Force. Final recommendation statement: cervical cancer: screening. U.S. preventive services task force. 2012. Available at: https://www.uspreventiveservicestaskforce.org/Page/Document/Recommendation StatementFinal/cervical-cancer-screening. Accessed June 27, 2018.
44. Abreu ALP, Souza RP, Gimenes F, et al. A review of methods for detect human Papillomavirus infection. Virology 2012;9:262.
45. Meites E, Kempe A, Markowitz LE. Use of a 2-dose schedule for human papillomavirus vaccination - updated recommendations of the advisory committee on immunization practices. MMWR Morb Mortal Wkly Rep 2016;65(49):1405–8.
46. Markowitz L, Liu G, Hariri S, et al. Prevalence of HPV after introduction of the vaccination program in the United States. Pediatrics 2016;137(3):e20151968.
47. Moosazadeh M, Haghshenas M, Mousavi T, et al. Efficacy of human papillomavirus l1 protein vaccines (Cervarix and Gardasil) in reducing the risk of cervical intraepithelial neoplasia: a meta-analysis. Int J Prev Med 2017;8(1):44–9.
48. Markowitz L. 2-dose human papillomavirus (HPV) vaccination schedules. Available at: http://www.cdc.gov/vaccines/acip/meetings/downloads/slides-2014-06/HPV-04- Markowitz.pdf. Accessed April 22, 2018.
49. Dobson SR, McNeil S, Dionne M, et al. Immunogenicity of 2 doses of HPV vaccine in younger adolescents vs 3 doses in young women: a randomized clinical trial. JAMA 2013;309(17):1793–802.
50. Lagheden C, Eklund C, Lamin H, et al. Nationwide comprehensive human papillomavirus (HPV) genotyping of invasive cervical cancer. Br J Cancer 2018; 118(10):1377–81.
51. Velentzis L, Caruana M, Simms K, et al. How will transitioning from cytology to HPV testing change the balance between the benefits and harms of cervical cancer screening? Estimates of the impact on cervical cancer, treatment rates and adverse obstetric outcomes in Australia, a high vaccination coverage country. Int J Cancer 2017;141(12):2410–22.

52. Patient information about GARDASIL® 9 (human papillomavirus 9-valent vaccine, recombinant) [package insert]. Whitehouse Station, NJ: Merck Sharp & Dohme Corp; 2016.

53. Garland S, Ault K, Gall S, et al. Pregnancy and infant outcomes in the clinical trials of a human papillomavirus type 6/11/16/18 vaccine. Obstet Gynecol 2009; 114(6):1179–88.

54. Habbema D, Weinmann S, Arbyn M, et al. Harms of cervical cancer screening in the United States and the Netherlands. Int J Cancer 2017;140(5):1215–22.

Colorectal Cancer Screening

Nikerson Geneve, DO[a], Daniel Kairys, MD[b],*, Bralin Bean, DO[a],
Tyler Provost, DO[a], Ron Mathew, DO[a], Nergess Taheri, DO[a]

KEYWORDS

- Colorectal cancer screening • Pathogenesis • Risk factors • Screening tests
- High-risk groups • Surveillance recommendations • Office practice

KEY POINTS

- Colorectal cancer can be reduced with appropriate implementation of an effective colorectal cancer screening program. Despite the wide availability of colorectal cancer screening tests, colorectal cancer screening remains low in the general population.
- There are 2 types of screening used in the United States for colorectal cancer screening: programmatic and opportunistic. The method used is based on the interaction between a patient and the health care provider.
- According to the US Preventive Services Task Force (USPSTF), screening for colorectal cancer should start at age 50 years and continue until age 75 years (category A recommendation). For adults aged 76 to 85 years, the decision to screen should be individualized, taking into account the patient's overall health and prior screening history (category C recommendation).
- The USPSTF does not recommend colorectal cancer screening for adults older than 85 years.
- Patient education is very important in an effective colorectal cancer screening program.

INTRODUCTION

Because colon cancer is among the leading causes of cancer in the United States, colon cancer prevention has become a very important topic of discussion for primary care physicians. Although mortality from colon cancer is preventable with appropriate screening, colorectal cancer screening rates remain below target levels in the general population. There are several factors to consider in colorectal cancer screening. Factors discussed in this article include the pathogenesis of colon cancer, risk factors, approaches to screening, available screening tests, and screening in high-risk groups. Considerations for office practice are also discussed.

The death rate from colorectal cancer has been declining in both men and women over the last several decades. Colorectal cancer screening is likely detecting

---

Disclosure Statement: The authors have nothing to disclose.
[a] Residency in Family Medicine, Lakeside Medical Center, 39200 Hooker Highway, Belle Glade, FL 33430, USA; [b] Department of General Surgery, Northern Light Maine Coast Hospital, 50 Union Street, Ellsworth, ME 04605, USA
* Corresponding author.
E-mail address: dbkairys@gmail.com

colorectal polyps earlier, when they can be removed before they can develop into cancers or when treatment improves outcomes. Research and treatment strategies have also improved; there now more than 1 million survivors of colorectal cancer in the United States.[1]

PATHOGENESIS OF COLON CARCINOMA
Adenoma-Carcinoma Sequence

As a scientific community, the current understanding of the pathogenesis of colon carcinoma describes what is known as the adenoma-carcinoma sequence as the primary way in which colon carcinoma develops. A basic understanding of this pathway demonstrates the necessity to screen for colon cancer because the pathologic progression allows for intervention and affects outcomes. The adenoma-carcinoma sequence describes the molecular means by which normal colonic mucosa progresses to an adenomatous polyp and then to carcinoma. Mutation to the adenomatous polyposis coli (APC) tumor suppressor gene marks the beginning of the sequence and leads to dysplasia of the normal colonic mucosa, placing it at risk for transformation into an adenoma. Note that germline mutations of this gene lead to familial adenomatous polyposis (FAP). Next, an activating mutation to K-ras, an oncogene, transforms the vulnerable, dysplastic mucosa into an adenomatous polyp. Finally, mutation to the p53 gene leads to the adenoma's conversion to carcinoma. Clinically, the slow development and growth of benign adenomatous polyps that eventually lead to carcinoma provides an opportunity to screen and prevent the development of colon carcinoma by way of secondary prevention.[2] Early identification and removal of polyps before they transition to cancerous tumors prevents many cases of cancer.

Much information is available regarding the functions of the genes involved in this pathway and the detailed mechanisms by which their mutations lead to colon carcinoma; these continue to be a topic of research.[3]

Right-sided Versus Left-Sided (Serrated Adenomas)

Polyps can occur within any section of the colon but it is helpful to differentiate right-sided versus left-sided. Adenomatous polyps occur significantly more frequently on the right compared with the left. It follows that right-sided polyps have a significantly higher potential for dysplasia and malignancy. Left-sided polyps are more frequently hyperplastic and benign in nature. Another type, serrated polyps, is a group of polyps that include the sessile serrated adenomas (SSAs), which are, as the name implies, flat, smooth, usually left-sided polyps that can be hidden by minimal stool or mucus. SSAs are often dysplastic with malignant potential. Due to their morphology, SSAs have increased potential to be missed or incompletely removed during colonoscopy and are, therefore, a significant source of colon carcinoma.[4]

RISK FACTORS FOR COLON CANCER
Family History

Having first-degree relatives with colorectal cancer increases the risk of developing cancer 2-fold. First-degree relatives include parent, child, or sibling. Risk is further increased with 2 first-degree relatives or 1 first-degree and 1 second-degree relative, or in those relatives diagnosed before the age of 50 years.[5]

Race

African Americans have the highest incidence of colorectal carcinomas than all other ethnic groups. More specifically, 20% higher than whites. Colorectal cancers in this ethnic group tend to occur in higher frequency in those who are younger than 50 years old. Therefore, screening in African Americans, as recommended by the American College of Gastroenterology (ACG), should begin at the age of 45 years.[6]

Gender

The incidence of colorectal mortality in men is 25% higher than in women. There is more proximal distribution of colorectal carcinomas and adenomas in women; therefore, flexible sigmoidoscopy may not be an adequate screening tool in women.[5]

Inflammatory Bowel Disease

Those with ulcerative colitis (UC) have increased risk depending on the extent, duration, and activity of disease. Those who have chronically active disease carry more risk than those who have quiescent disease. There is a 0.5% risk per year for those with duration of 10 to 20 years, then a 1% increase for every year beyond that. Pancolitis itself has a 5-fold to 10-fold increase, this usually occurs about 8 to 10 years after it has been diagnosed. Left-sided UC also has high risk, about a 3-fold increase.[7]

By the third decade of life, those with UC will have a 30% increase in the risk of malignancy. There is increased risk with UC and primary sclerosing cholangitis. Further risk of malignancy with UC depends on pseudopolyps and strictures. The mean age for diagnosis of malignancy in UC is 43 years old. Crohn disease has similar risk of colon cancer as those with UC. Surveillance should occur in those who have greater than one-third of the colon involved. The mean age for diagnosis of malignancy is 55 years.[7]

Other Cancer and Colon Cancer Risk

Early abdominal radiation in childhood and adolescence has been associated with subsequent gastrointestinal (GI) neoplasms, especially colorectal cancers. For those who received 30 Gy or more of abdominal radiation, colonoscopy is recommended every 5 years. Screening should begin 10 years after radiation or at the age of 35 years, whichever is later.[5] Those who have had external radiation treatment for prostate cancer have the same risk for colon cancer as those with a family history of colonic adenomas. Thus there is a more frequent association with colorectal cancers.[5] Endometrial cancer is the second most common cancer associated with Lynch syndrome, thus there is an associated 80% lifetime risk for developing colorectal cancer. Women diagnosed with endometrial cancer before age 50 years have an even greater risk. Most colon cancers associated with endometrial cancer are right-sided and occur in women age 51 to 65 years.[8]

Human Immunodeficiency Virus

There is increased risk, about 30-fold, for anal squamous carcinoma in patients with human immunodeficiency virus (HIV). As for all other colorectal cancers, there is no increased risk. HIV-infected individuals have equal risk to non-HIV infected individuals.[8]

Genetic Syndromes

FAP is associated with numerous colonic adenomas, which usually appear during childhood. The symptoms approximated appear at age 16 years and account for 1% of colorectal cancers. About 90% of those with untreated FAP will have colonic cancer by the age of 45 years. There is an association with the APC gene on chromosome 5. The Ashkenazi Jewish population with FAP have a further 1.5-fold to 2-fold increased risk of colon cancer.[5]

MUTYH-associated polyposis is an autosomal recessive syndrome from the biallelic germline mutations in the base excision repair gene mutY homolog. Lynch syndrome is an autosomal dominant caused by a DNA mismatch repair (MMR) gene. About 3% of all colonic adenocarcinomas are associated with Lynch syndrome. There is early onset, with mean age of 48 years, and some patients have onset as early as their 20s. Most lesions are right-sided, about 70% will arise proximal to the splenic flexure.[5]

SPECIFIC SCREENING TESTS

Colonoscopy is among the most sensitive and specific of all the screening tests. It is 80% to 95% sensitive and nearly 95% to 100% specific. The added advantage is that polyp removal is possible during the procedure. However, there is the associated risk with conscious sedation and electrolyte abnormalities due to the bowel preparation. Furthermore, there are risks of perforation and bleeding that occur rarely. The benefits of screening outweigh the risks. As previously stated, examinations should start at age 50 years, then every 10 years, unless otherwise indicated owing to higher risk or other criteria.[9]

Fecal immunochemical (FIT) tests detect only globin and are said to be more specific than other tests that screen for fecal occult blood. This is because globin is digested in the upper GI system, so bleeding is more specific to the lower GI system. This is an annual test. Specificity is 77% and sensitivity is 94%.[10] Cologuard (Exact Sciences Corporation, Madison, WI) is a test that combines stool for DNA mutations and methylation markers using a gene-amplification technique, as well as hemoglobin, with FIT. Sensitivity is 92% for detecting stages 1 to 4 colon cancer and 94% for detecting early stages 1 to 2. Specificity is 87%. Its more sensitive than FIT but less specific.[11]

Computed tomographic (CT) colonoscopy takes multiple images of the colon that are thinly sliced and uses a computer to construct them into a 2-dimensional or a 3-dimensional image. It is performed every 5 years. It can be 67% to 94% sensitive and 96% to 98% specific for colorectal cancer detection.

Flex sigmoidoscopy is mainly specific for left-sided cancers and can be done every 5 years. This, however, is not effective in women who tend to have right-sided cancers. The sensitivity is 67% but combined with FIT it is 75% to 89%.[12]

Capsule colonoscopy uses a tiny camera that is embedded into 2 ends of an ingested capsule to take images as it travels through the colon. It requires more rigorous bowel prep than colonoscopies. In the United States this is only approved for those who have had an incomplete colonoscopy, not as a stand-alone screening test. The sensitivity and specificity were 64% and 84% for detecting 6 mm polyps or advanced adenomas.[13]

Septin 9 DNA is hypermethylated in colorectal cancer but not in normal colon tissue. This assay is for average-risk patients who refuse other screening methods. Positive tests should be followed by colonoscopy. It has a 27% false-positive rate and some new ones have as low as 4.7 false-positive rates. It is 70% sensitive and 90% specific.[14]

Approaches to Screening

There are 2 types of screening approaches used for colorectal cancer screening: programmatic and opportunistic. Programmatic screening is a system-wide approach that offers screening to a population of people with a predetermined approach. Potential advantages of programmatic screening include systematic offers of screening, reduction of overscreening, superior monitoring of quality, and systematic follow-up of results.[15] The United States has no national program for colorectal cancer screening, whereas other countries with national health plans are experimenting with these programs.[16] The United States has been successful in increasing colorectal cancer screening rates and reducing mortality using an opportunistic approach. Colorectal cancer screening reduced the incidence of colorectal cancer by 3% to 4% per year and by 30% overall in the first decade of this century. Awareness of colorectal cancer and insurance coverage of screening are likely reflective of the high rates of screening. Relying on opportunistic screening may allow preference for colorectal cancer screening owing to compliance with tests that need to be repeated at specified short intervals, which is more challenging.[15]

With opportunistic screening, providers may use several broad strategies to offer screening to patients. When patients are offered both colonoscopy and fecal occult blood testing, more patients undergo screening. In 1 study, offering additional screening methods, such as 5 choices, did not improve compliance compared with offering 2 screening options. Physicians can limit options to 2 or 3, while engaging in shared decision-making with patients, offering additional options in the event a patient declines.[15]

A sequential approach is recommended by the ACG and the American Society for Gastrointestinal Endoscopy, with colonoscopy being the first choice. Providers place a high emphasis on the efficacy of colonoscopy in preventing colorectal cancer and less emphasis on the risks associated with colonoscopy. Another option often used in the sequential testing method is to offer patients a FIT test as the initial screening test.[17]

A risk-stratified approach uses evidence that represents a wide range of risk that can be estimated based on demographics and risk factors that include older age, male gender, obesity, diabetes, and cigarette smoking. The goal is to find patients at risk for precancerous lesions who would benefit most from colonoscopy. Risk stratification is poorly accepted owing to the limited accuracy in discriminating high and low prevalence groups. Recent models increase the accuracy of high-risk and low-risk groups for advanced adenomas. No studies are available that compare compliance or outcomes with a risk-stratified approach to multiple options or sequential approaches.[17]

The US Multi-Service Task Force on Colorectal Cancer considers each of these approaches as reasonable when offered in an opportunistic setting. No evidence exists that suggests any approach compared with another. Patients should know that if they do not have a colonoscopy for their screening method, they will need to undergo colonoscopy for further evaluation if their initial screening test is positive.[17]

SCREENING IN HIGH-RISK GROUPS

There is a general consensus among the different professional organizations that those with certain red flags are at an increased risk of developing colon polyps or cancer. High-risk patients may have characteristics such as a personal or family history of FAP or hereditary nonpolyposis colorectal cancer (HNPCC), a personal history of colorectal polyps or cancers, or have an associated inflammatory bowel disease (IBD), such as Crohn disease or UC. Patients with a family history of colorectal cancer (a first-degree relative with early-onset colorectal cancer or multiple first-degree relatives with the disease) can be screened more frequently starting at a younger age with colonoscopy. Screening for the different high-risk groups can be generally divided into 2 categories: familial colorectal cancer syndromes or IBDs.[6]

Lynch syndrome, also known as HNPCC, is the most common form of hereditary colon cancer. It is inherited in an autosomal dominant fashion caused by defective

MMR proteins. The Amsterdam Criteria is a widely regarded means by which to screen for HNPCC and consists of the following:

- Three or more family members with a confirmed diagnosis of colorectal cancer, 1 whom is a first-degree (parent, child, sibling) relative of the other 2
- Two successive affected generations
- One or more colon cancers diagnosed at younger than 50 years of age
- FAP has been excluded.

Familial colorectal cancer type, also known as syndrome X, is a type of HNPCC that differs from HNPCC in that there is no mutation in the MMR gene, so the tumors produced are microsatellite stable.[18]

FAP is an inherited, non–sex-linked, autosomal dominant disease accounting for approximately 1% of all colorectal cancers. It is caused by mutations in the tumor-suppressor *APC* gene, located on chromosome 5 (5q21–q22), or in the *MUTYH* gene, which is located on chromosome 1 (1p34.3–p32.1). It is known for the prevalent, progressive development of hundreds or thousands of adenomatous polyps located throughout the entire colon.[19] Gardner syndrome is considered a subset of FAP.

IBDs are a collective of inflammatory conditions that affect the small intestine and colon and are characterized by 2 principal types: UC and Crohn disease. They are associated with an increased risk of colorectal cancer due to their duration but have key differences on their causation. UC, in terms of its duration and extent in primarily affecting the rectum and colon (left-sided vs the whole colon) is thought to have double the risk toward colorectal cancer compared with Crohn disease. Crohn disease can affect the mouth, esophagus, stomach, small intestine, colon, and anus.[19]

Surveillance Recommendations

Screening and surveillance programs involve visually examining the intestinal tract to check its healthy condition (via colonoscopy of flexible sigmoidoscopy) and allow earlier detection of polyposis before it becomes life-threatening. In a high-risk group, certain factors are taken into account, such as the genetic predispositions discussed earlier, family history, and age considerations. These factors dictate when to undertake screening, particularly when either a genetic test has confirmed the risk or a genetic test has not been undertaken for any reason so that the actual risk is unknown. Although the best age to initiate and discontinue screening, as well as the frequency and preferred screening method, can vary from person to person, as well as whether they are classified in an average-risk or high-risk group, many organizations have published guidelines concerning screening and surveillance for colorectal cancer. In particular are the American Cancer Society, US Multi-Society Task Force on Colorectal Cancer (**Tables 1** and **2**), American College of Radiology, US Preventive Services Task Force, American College of Physicians, and ACG.

A jointly issued recommendation by the American Cancer Society, American College of Radiology, and the US Multi-Society Task Force on Colorectal Cancer (including the American Gastroenterological Association, ACG, and American Society for Gastrointestinal Endoscopy) recommended screening for colorectal cancer and adenomatous polyps starting at age 50 years in asymptomatic (average-risk) men and women.[20] They prioritized the use of any of the following tests: flexible sigmoidoscopy every 5 years, colonoscopy every 10 years, double-contrast barium enema every 5 years, and CT colonography every 5 years. In 2017, the US Multi-Society

Table 1
American Cancer Society guidelines on screening and surveillance for the early detection of colorectal adenomas and cancer in people at increased risk or high risk

Risk Factors			
Risk Category	When to Test	Recommended Tests	Comment
People with small rectal hyperplastic polyps	Same age as those at average risk	Colonoscopy or other screening options at same intervals as for those at average risk	Those with hyperplastic polyposis syndrome are at increased risk for adenomatous polyps and cancer and should have more intensive follow-up.
People with 1 or 2 small (no more than 1 cm) tubular adenomas with low-grade dysplasia	5–10 y after the polyps are removed	Colonoscopy	Time between tests should be based on other factors such as prior colonoscopy findings, family history, and patient and doctor preferences.
People with 3–10 adenomas, a large (at least 1 cm) adenoma, or any adenomas with high-grade dysplasia or villous features	3 y after the polyps are removed	Colonoscopy	Adenomas must have been completely removed. If colonoscopy is normal or shows only 1 or 2 small tubular adenomas with low-grade dysplasia, future colonoscopies can be done every 5 y.
People with more than 10 adenomas on a single examination	Within 3 y after the polyps are removed	Colonoscopy	Doctor should consider possible genetic syndrome (eg, FAP or Lynch syndrome).
People with sessile adenomas that are removed in pieces	2–6 mo after adenoma removal	Colonoscopy	If entire adenoma has been removed, further testing should be based on doctor's judgment.
Increased Risk: People Who Have Had Colorectal Cancer			
Risk Category	When to Test	Recommended Tests	Comment
People diagnosed with colon or rectal cancer	At time of colorectal surgery, or can be 3–6 months post surgery in the case of emergent resections (in the absence of unresectable metastatic disease)	Colonoscopy to look at the entire colon and remove all polyps	If the tumor is obstructing at time of diagnosis, CT colonography or double contrast barium enema may be done to examine the remainder of the colonic mucosa prior to surgery

(continued on next page)

Table 1
(continued)

Increased Risk: People Who Have Had Colorectal Cancer

Risk Category	When to Test	Recommended Tests	Comment
People who have had colon or rectal cancer removed by surgery	1 y after cancer resection (or 1 y after colonoscopy to make sure the rest of the colon or rectum was clear)	Colonoscopy	If normal, repeat in 3 y. If normal, repeat test every 5 y. Time between tests may be shorter if polyps are found or there is reason to suspect Lynch syndrome. After low anterior resection for rectal cancer, examinations of the rectum may be done every 3–6 mo for the first 2–3 y to look for signs of recurrence.

Increased Risk: People with a Family History

Risk Category	Age to Start Testing	Recommended Tests	Comment
Colorectal cancer or adenomatous polyps in any first-degree relative before age 60 y, or in 2 or more first-degree relatives at any age (if not a hereditary syndrome)	Age 40 y, or 10 y before the youngest case in the immediate family, whichever is earlier	Colonoscopy	Every 5 y
Colorectal cancer or adenomatous polyps in any first-degree relative aged 60 y or older, or in at least 2 second-degree relatives at any age	Age 40 y	Same test options as for those at average risk	Same test intervals as for those at average risk

High Risk

Risk Category	Age to Start Testing	Recommended Tests	Comment
FAP diagnosed by genetic testing, or suspected FAP without genetic testing	Age 10–12 y	Yearly flexible sigmoidoscopy to look for signs of FAP; counseling to consider genetic testing if it has not been done	If genetic test is positive, removal of colon (colectomy) should be considered.

(continued on next page)

Table 1 *(continued)*			
High Risk			
Risk Category	**Age to Start Testing**	**Recommended Tests**	**Comment**
Lynch syndrome (hereditary nonpolyposis colorectal cancer or HNPCC), or at increased risk of Lynch syndrome based on family history without genetic testing	Age 20–25 y, or 10 y before the youngest case in the immediate family	Colonoscopy every 1–2 y; counseling to consider genetic testing if it has not been done	Genetic testing should be offered to first-degree relatives of people found to have Lynch syndrome mutations by genetic tests. It should also be offered if 1 of the first 3 of the modified Bethesda criteria is met.
IBD: • Chronic UC • Crohn disease	Cancer risk begins to be significant 8 y after the onset of pancolitis (involvement of entire large intestine), or 12–15 y after the onset of left-sided colitis	Colonoscopy every 1–2 y with biopsies for dysplasia	These people are best referred to a center with experience in the surveillance and management of IBD.

Adapted from Levin B, Lieberman DA, McFarland B, et al. Screening and surveillance for the early detection of colorectal cancer and adenomatous polyps, 2008: a joint guideline from the American Cancer Society, the US Multi-Society Task Force on Colorectal Cancer, and the American College of Radiology. Gastroenterology 2008;134(5):1588–9; with permission.

Task Force on Colorectal Cancer issued updated screening recommendations that divide screening tests into 3 tiers, based on effectiveness:

- Tier 1: colonoscopy every 10 years, annual FIT
- Tier 2: CT colonography every 5 years, FIT-fecal DNA every 3 years, or flexible sigmoidoscopy every 5 to 10 years
- Tier 3: capsule colonoscopy every 5 years (septin 9 testing is not recommended).[21]

For patients at average risk, testing with a tier 1 test should begin at age 45 years for African Americans and at age 50 years for patients of all other races. Patients with a family history of colorectal cancer or advanced adenoma diagnosed before age 60 years in 1 first-degree relative or at any age in 2 first-degree relatives should begin screening with a colonoscopy when they are 10 years younger than the youngest age at diagnosis of a first-degree relative. This group should be tested every 5 years. Patients with 1 first-degree relative with colorectal cancer, advanced adenoma, or an advanced serrated lesion diagnosed at age 60 or older have the same screening recommendations as average-risk patients:

- Guaiac-based fecal occult blood test, every year
- FIT, every year
- FIT-DNA, every 1 or 3 years
- Colonoscopy, every 10 years
- CT colonography, every 5 years

Table 2
Screening high-risk patients for colorectal cancer

Risk Category	Age to Begin	Recommended Test	Comment
HNPCC or risk for HNPCC (Lynch Syndrome)	Age 20–25 y, or 10 y before the age at onset of youngest affected family member	Colonoscopy, counseling for genetic testing	Every 1–2 y Genetic testing should be offered to first-degree relatives of persons with a known DNA-MMR gene defect or with 1 of the first 3 Bethesda criteria.
FAP or suspected FAP	Age 10–12 y	Annual flexible sigmoidoscopy, counseling for genetic testing if showing polyps	Colectomy should be considered for positive genetic testing.
Personal history of 3–10 adenomas, or 1 adenoma >1 cm, or any adenoma with villous features or high-grade dysplasia	3 y after the initial polypectomy	Colonoscopy	Adenomas require compete excision. If the follow-up is normal, the next examination should be in 5 y. Presence of >10 adenomas should raise suspicion of a familial syndrome.
Personal history of <3 adenomas with low-grade dysplasia	5–10 y after the initial polypectomy	Colonoscopy	Examination interval should be based on other clinical factors, such as prior findings, family history, or endoscopist or patient preference.
Personal history of colorectal cancer	1 y after resection	Colonoscopy	Patients should undergo high-quality preoperative clearance. Follow-up after normal examinations should be extended to 3 y and then to 5 y.
Family history of adenomas or cancer in a first-degree relative <60 y of age or in 2 first-degree relatives at any age	Age 40 y, or 10 y before the age at onset of youngest affected family member	Colonoscopy	Every 5 y

(continued on next page)

Table 2 (*continued*)			
Risk Category	**Age to Begin**	**Recommended Test**	**Comment**
Family history of adenomas or cancer in 1 first-degree relative >60 y of age or in 2 second-degree relatives with cancer	Age 40 y	Colonoscopy	Screening should be initiated at an earlier age. Intervals are based on findings or on the average-risk patient.
IBD, Crohn disease, or chronic UC	8 y after the onset of pancolitis, or 12–15 y after the onset of left-sided colitis	Colonoscopies with random 4-quadrant biopsies every 10 cm for dysplasia	Screening should be offered every 1–2 y, and patients are best referred to a center with experience in the surveillance and management of IBD.

Abbreviations: FS, flexible sigmoidoscopy.

From Maxwell PJ, Isenberg GA. Tumors of the colon and rectum. In: Kellerman RD, Bope ET, editors. Conn's current therapy 2018. Philadelphia: Elsevier; 2018. p. 248–52; with permission.

- Flexible sigmoidoscopy, every 5 years
- Flexible sigmoidoscopy with FIT; sigmoidoscopy every 10 years, with FIT every year.

Colonoscopy screening should be discontinued in patients aged 75 years or older with prior negative screening tests, those whose life expectancy is less than 10 years, or in those 85 years or older without prior screening.[22]

According to the ACG, there is a distinction between screening tests for cancer prevention and cancer detection. Preventive tests are preferred compared with those that only detect, particularly colonoscopy every 10 years (starting at age 45 in African Americans and at age 50 years in other races). For those who decline colonoscopy or another cancer prevention test, the preferred cancer detection test is FIT, which is conducted annually. Alternative cancer detection tests recommended by ACG guidelines are flexible sigmoidoscopy every 5 to 10 years and CT colonography every 5 years (replacing double-contrast barium enema as the radiographic screening alternative for patients who decline colonoscopy). Additional cancer tests in the ACG guidelines include the annual Hemoccult Sensa (Beckham Coulter Life Sciences, Indianapolis, IN), or fecal DNA, testing every 3 years. Additional recommendations by the ACG state that patients with 1 first-degree relative diagnosed with colorectal cancer or advanced adenoma at age 60 years or older are considered average-risk. Those with 1 first-degree relative diagnosed with colorectal cancer or advanced adenoma before age 60 years, or those with 2 first-degree relatives with colorectal cancer or advanced adenomas, are recommended to get colonoscopy every 5 years, beginning at age 40 years, or at 10 years younger than the age at diagnosis of the youngest affected relative.[22]

CONSIDERATIONS FOR OFFICE PRACTICE

Because it is among the most common forms of cancer diagnosis in the United States, most organizations recommend that average-risk individuals begin screenings for colorectal cancer at 50 years of age.[23] Unfortunately, despite the widely available methods of colorectal cancer screening, screening rates in the general population remains low. However, with the variety of colorectal cancer screening measures available, the question of what is the best screening tests for colorectal cancer screening test is often posed by patients in the office practice setting. The best screening tests are any that get done. However, there are several factors that come in to play when trying to improve screening implementation for colorectal cancer screening. A key factor is the role of the physician. "A recommendation from a physician is the most influential factor in determining whether a patient is screened for colorectal cancer."[24] In addition, according to Fleming and colleagues,[25] the most effective mode of outreach for colorectal cancer screening is when the patient has an in-person conversation with a clinician about FIT testing and receives the FIT test during the visit.

Other options include open-access colonoscopy. This model connects the gastroenterology practice directly with the patient and eliminates the need for preprocedure office visits in selected patients. The purpose of open-access colonoscopy is to provide an efficient means to meet the growing need for colorectal cancer screening. The challenge in this setting is effective communication between the primary care physician and the gastroenterology practice in regard to the outcome of the colonoscopy and necessary follow-up. Assuring proper procedure indication and minimizing medical legal risks can also be a challenge in this model.[26]

Frequently, the questions patients ask involve the follow-up care of the survivor of colorectal cancer. Consequently, follow-up care of the colorectal cancer screening survivor is a very important topic of discussion. "Several organization including the American Cancer Society recommend intensive postoperative surveillance based on a conservative interpretation of the available evidence. Beginning four to six weeks after the potentialy curative resection, follow up should occur every 3–6 months for the first 2–3 years, then every six months for a total of 5 years. Carcinoembryonic antigen (CEA) testing is recommended at each visit."[27] Colorectal cancer survivors should be screened for other cancers according to the same guidelines used for average-risk persons. This approach is similar to health promotion for the general population. This includes evidence-based weight loss interventions and exercising the recommended 150 minutes per week. Smoking cessation is of tremendous value in reducing the overall cancer-related mortality rates. Another consideration is the role of aspirin. Currently, the US Preventive Task Force recommends aspirin for primary prevention in a select group of patients. "If no contraindications exists, daily low-dose aspirin for colorectal cancer survivors with a life expectancy of at least 10 years is reasonable in addition to other recurrence prevention strategies."[27] Because of the complexity of the management of surveillance of colorectal cancer, as well as its potential complications, care coordination involving an oncology team can be of great use for both the patient and the primary care physician.

The cost-effectiveness of colonoscopy often comes up. Kingsley and colleagues[28] note that there are issues of overuse of colonoscopies, which can be because of endoscopist preference, patient preference, or inadequate bowel preparation. Inadequate bowel preparation results in colonoscopy being repeated every 7.8 years in average-risk patients instead of 10 years. This results in colonoscopy being performed much more frequently than is actually necessary. Education plays a very important role in curbing this overutilization. Both the gastroenterology office and the primary care physician need to educate patients on adequate bowel preparation. Kingsley and colleagues[28] concluded that "screening colonoscopy is not a cost effective strategy when compared with fecal immunochemical test, as long as the inadequate bowel preparation rate is greater than 13%." This further emphasizes the tremendous role that primary care physicians have in patient education for colorectal cancer screening.

Tables 1 and **2** provide guidance on screening and surveillance in those groups considered to be high-risk for colorectal cancer.[21]

REFERENCES

1. American Cancer Society. Cancer facts & figures 2018. Atlanta (GA): American Cancer Society; 2018. Available at: https://www.cancer.org/cancer/colon-rectal-cancer/about/key-statistics.html. Accessed November 11, 2018.

2. Bond JH. Clinical evidence for the adenoma-carcinoma sequence, and the management of patients with colorectal adenomas. Semin Gastrointest Dis 2000; 11(4):176–84. Available at: http://europepmc.org/abstract/med/11057945.

3. Leslie A, Carey FA, Pratt NR, et al. The colorectal adenoma–carcinoma sequence. Br J Surg 2002;89:845–60. Available at: http://onlinelibrary.wiley.com/doi/10.1046/j.1365-2168.2002.02120.x/epdf.

4. Qumseya BJ, Coe S, Wallace MB. The effect of polyp location and patient gender on the presence of dysplasia in colonic polyps. Clin Transl Gastroenterol 2012; 3(7):e20. Available at: https://www.ncbi.nlm.nih.gov/pmc/articles/PMC3412677/.

5. Macrae F. Colorectal cancer: epidemiology, risk factors, and protective factors. 2018. Available at: https://www.uptodate.com/contents/colorectal-cancer-epidemiology-risk-factors-and-protective-factors#!. Accessed April 15, 2018.

6. Rex DK, Johnson DA, Anderson JC, et al. American College of Gastroenterology guidelines for colorectal cancer screening 2009 [corrected]. Am J Gastroenterol 2009;104:739–50.

7. Shergill A, Odze R, Farraye F. Surveillance and management of dysplasia in patients with inflammatory bowel disease. 2018. Available at: https://www.uptodate.com/contents/surveillance-and-management-of-dysplasia-in-patients-with-inflammatory-bowel-disease?sectionName=Crohn disease&anchor=H2089418339&source=see_link#H2089418339. Accessed April 15, 2018.

8. Sigel K, Dubrow R, Silverberg M, et al. Cancer screening in patients infected with HIV. Curr HIV/AIDS Rep 2011;8(3):142–52.

9. NIH (2017) Colorectal Cancer Mortality Projections. Available at: https://cisnet.cancer.gov/projections/colorectal/screening.php. Accessed April 15, 2018.

10. Robertson DJ, Lee JK, Boland CR, et al. Recommendations on fecal immunochemical testing to screen for colorectal neoplasia: a consensus statement by the US Multi-Society Task Force on Colorectal Cancer. Gastroenterology 2017; 152(5). https://doi.org/10.1053/j.gastro.2016.08.053.

11. Brown T. FDA panel unanimously backs Cologuard colorectal cancer test. New York: MedScape; 2014. Available at: https://www.medscape.com/viewarticle/822709.

12. Niedermaier T, Weigl K, Hoffmeister M, et al. Diagnostic performance of flexible sigmoidoscopy combined with fecal immunochemical test in colorectal cancer screening: meta-analysis and modeling. Eur J Epidemiol 2017;32:481.

13. Doubeni C. Tests for screening for colorectal cancer: Stool tests, radiologic imaging and endoscopy. 2017. Available at: https://www.uptodate.com/contents/tests-for-screening-for-colorectal-cancer-stool-tests-radiologic-imaging-and-endoscopy?search=fit test&source=search_result&selectedTitle=1~150&usage_type=default&display_rank=1#H6. Accessed April 15, 2018.

14. Molnár B, Tóth K, Barták BK, et al. Plasma methylated septin 9: a colorectal cancer screening marker. Expert Rev Mol Diagn 2014;15(2):171–84.

15. Levin TR, Corley DA, Jensen CD, et al. Effects of organized colorectal cancer screening on cancer incidence and mortality in a large, community-based population. Gastroenterology 2018;155(5):1383–91.e5.

16. Telford JJ. Canadian guidelines for colorectal cancer screening. Can J Gastroenterol 2011;25(9):479–81.

17. Rex DK, Boland CR, Dominitz JA, et al. Colorectal cancer screening: recommendations for physicians and patients from the U.S. Multi-Society Task Force on Colorectal Cancer. Am J Gastroenterol 2017;112:1016–30.

18. Lindor NM, Rabe K, Petersen GM, et al. Lower cancer incidence in Amsterdam-I criteria families without mismatch repair deficiency: familial colorectal cancer type X. JAMA 2005;293(16):1979–85.

19. Maxwell PJ, Isenberg GA. Tumors of the colon and rectum. In: Bope ET, Kellerman RD, editors. Conn's current therapy 2018. Atlanta (GA): Elsevier; 2018. p. 248–52.

20. Berger E, Sherrod A, Alteri R, et al. American Cancer Society recommendations for colorectal cancer early detection. 2018. Available at: https://www.cancer.org/cancer/colon-rectal-cancer/detection-diagnosis-staging/acs-recommendations.html. April 23, 2018.

21. Final recommendation statement: colorectal cancer: screening. U.S. Preventive Services Task Force. 2017. Available at: https://www.uspreventiveservicestaskforce.org/Page/Document/RecommendationStatementFinal/colorectal-cancer-screening2. April 23, 2018.

22. Cabebe EC, Espat NJ. Colorectal cancer guidelines. 2017. Available at: https://emedicine.medscape.com/article/2500006-overview. Accessed April 23, 2018.

23. Wilkins T, McMechan D, Talukder A, et al. Colorectal cancer screening and surveillance in individuals at increased risk. Am Fam Physician 2018;97:111–6.

24. Sarfaty M, Richard W. How to increase colorectal cancer screening rates. CA Cancer J Clin 2007;57(6):354–66.

25. Fleming TJ, Benitez MG, Weintraub MLR. Evaluating the effectivenesss of one on one conversations to increase colorectal cancer screening in a community based clinical setting. J Am Osteopath Assoc 2018;118(1):26–33.

26. Pike IM. Open access endoscopy. Gastrointest Endosc Clin N Am 2006;12(4):709–17.

27. Burgers K, Moore C, Bednash L. Care of the colorectal cancer survivor. Am Fam Physician 2018;97:331–6.

28. Kingsley J, Karanth S, Revere FL, et al. Cost effectiveness of screening colonoscopy depends on adequate bowel preparation rates - a modeling study. PLoS One 2016;11(12):e0167452.

Prostate Cancer Screening

Shared Decision-Making for Screening and Treatment

Russ Blackwelder, MD, MDiv, CMD[a,b,*], Alexander Chessman, MD[a]

KEYWORDS

- Prostate cancer • Screening • Cancer prevention • Men's health

KEY POINTS

- Shared decision-making about prostate cancer screening is recommended for men 55 to 69 years of age, according to the US Preventive Services Task Force.
- Younger men at higher risk, such as African American men, may also be good candidates for shared decision-making.
- As men age, screening increases the likelihood of harm and detection of clinically insignificant disease; therefore screening should end at age 70 years.
- Prostate cancer remains a major cause of worldwide morbidity, and more research on prevention and screening is needed.

INTRODUCTION

Prostate cancer has generated great controversy over the past few years, as reflected in the title of the editorial "Screening for prostate cancer—the controversy that refuses to die."[1] From stories in local media to conversations at the bedside, sorting through the arguments about screening for prostate cancer with the prostate-specific antigen (PSA) test and varied risks and benefits of treatment remains an evolving topic.

The use of PSA in screening for prostate cancer emerged in the 1980s; however, large sets of peer-reviewed data to inform decision-making were not available in the literature until 2009.[2] Although prostate cancer is common, sorting through what determines high-risk disease and weighing the benefits versus risks of intervention remain significant challenges for primary care providers.[3]

Although most recommendations encourage shared decision-making with patients for prostate cancer screening, finding the time for these discussions in a busy practice

Disclosure: The authors have nothing to disclose.
[a] Department of Family Medicine, MUSC, 5 Charleston Center, Suite 263, MSC #192, Charleston, SC 29425-0192, USA; [b] The Village at Summerville, 201 West 9th North Street, Summerville, SC 29483, USA
* Corresponding author. 5 Charleston Center, Suite 263, MSC #192, Charleston, SC 29425-0192, USA
E-mail address: blackwr@musc.edu

Prim Care Clin Office Pract 46 (2019) 149–155
https://doi.org/10.1016/j.pop.2018.10.012   **primarycare.theclinics.com**
0095-4543/19/© 2018 Elsevier Inc. All rights reserved.

is difficult, particularly because new evidence continues to add to the complexity of this conversation. This article reviews current knowledge about prostate cancer: its clinical presentation, epidemiology, the risks and benefits of screening, and therapy decisions.

CLINICAL DESCRIPTION OF DISEASE

Inferior to the bladder and surrounding the urethra, the prostate is responsible for contributing to semen production. Most often adenocarcinoma, prostate cancer is the most commonly diagnosed cancer and the second leading cause of cancer death in American men.[4] Before the late twentieth century, digital rectal examination (DRE) was the primary means of detecting prostate disease; however, this changed with the advent of PSA testing. DRE has a high rate of performer variability and, once a mass if felt, it can indicate more advanced cancer. This test was initially developed for prostate cancer surveillance; however, it was soon also used as a screening test.[5] As diagnosis of prostate cancer increased, treatment options and algorithms have continued to evolve. With the advent of prostate cancer screening with PSA testing came the advent of overdiagnosis of prostate cancers that are not life-threatening. Estimates are that for every death averted from prostate cancer screening, there are an additional 26 cases diagnosed.[6]

Though sensitivity and specificity for PSA testing depends on the threshold used, at a cutoff of 4.0 ng/mL the sensitivity is 20.5% and specificity is 93.8% for histologically positive prostate specimens.[7] Complicating factors even more is the challenge in determining which histologically positive prostate biopsies will lead to clinically significant disease. The Gleason score is the sum of the grading of the 2 most prevalent pathologic patterns seen on biopsy, each pattern rated from 1 to 5, with 5 being the most aggressive. A score of 6 or below is low risk, 7 is typically considered intermediate risk, and 8 or above is high risk. After diagnosis of prostate cancer is made, several algorithms can help to determine the best treatment options. The biopsy cores were previously taken in sextants of the prostate gland for a total of 6 samples; however, the current standard requires 10 to 12 tissue samples.[3]

PSA testing has a high false-positive rate, increased by factors such as prostatitis, ejaculation, trauma, and recent instrumentation. PSA testing also has a high rate of false negatives. Several options have been attempted to help predict clinically significant disease. PSA velocity, free PSA, protein-bound PSA, and PSA density have all been measured and studied but these means still lack clear evidence pertaining to their usefulness.[5]

With the advent of PSA testing, the lifetime risk of prostate cancer diagnosis increased from 9% in 1985 to 16% in 2007.[5] Treatment of prostate cancer is not without significant harms, most notably in sexual function and continence. Radical prostatectomy may have higher rates of harm versus external beam radiation therapy (EBRT) and active surveillance.[8] EBRT also carries risks of bowel irritation. EBRT and brachytherapy carry risks of urinary irritation and obstruction.[9]

EPIDEMIOLOGY

Prostate cancer is common. Outside of skin cancer, this cancer is the most frequently diagnosed cancer in the United States. It is the most common cancer diagnosed in men in the United States. Prostate cancer is the third leading cause of cancer-related deaths. Western, developed countries, where screening is more prevalent, have a higher incidence rate of prostate cancer than developing nations. There was an increase in the prevalence of prostate cancer with the advent of the serum PSA test. In many countries, such as the United States, the diagnosis of this type of cancer is greatly depends on the effort spent to detect the disease.[10]

Autopsy studies reveal a high rate of clinically undetected and incidental prostate cancer, a rate that increases with age. Combining studies from different countries, Jahn and colleagues[11] found prostate cancer in 36% of white men and 51% of African American men aged 70 to 79 years.

The cause is unknown. Family history increases risk. It is estimated that about 9% of prostate cancer may be hereditary because the presence of prostate cancer in one's father or 3 brothers increases the age-specific hazard ratio by 2.1 or 17.7, respectively.[12]

Black ancestry, perhaps West African ancestry, also seems to be a risk factor. Though white men have had a decreasing incidence and mortality from prostate cancer since 1991, African American men have not experienced a commensurate decrease. A study compared rates of cancer incidence, prevalence, and mortality in countries that were affected in the past by the transatlantic slave trade, finding similar patterns in the Caribbean Islands, United Kingdom, to the pattern for US black men. This evidence supports the theory that Africans taken into slavery brought increased risk with their genome.[13]

SCREENING GUIDELINES

Screening guidelines recommend shared decision-making with the patient, particularly sharing the risks and benefits of serum PSA testing. The US Preventive Services Task Force (USPSTF) recommends against PSA-based screening for prostate cancer for men aged 70 years and older. For men aged 55 to 69 years, the clinician should inform the patient about potential risks and benefits of screening, including the modest benefit of reduced risk for dying from prostate cancer balanced against the harms of screening. The patient should, however, understand the side effects of treatment, including incontinence and sexual dysfunction. Potential harm also includes false-positive PSA levels that lead to unnecessary, further testing and overtreatment.[14]

A Cochrane review conducted a meta-analysis of 5 studies and found no benefit to screening in reducing prostate cancer-related mortality.[15] Only 1 study found a benefit to screening the predefined subgroup of men aged 55 to 69 years of age. The European Randomized Study of Screening for Prostate Cancer (ERSPC) study focused on men aged 55 to 69 years in 8 European countries. The investigators found that 781 men would need to be screened to prevent 1 additional death from prostate cancer during a median follow-up duration of 13 years.[16] **Table 1** is taken from the USPSTF final recommendation and summarizes the outcomes based on screening 1000 men.

PREVENTION RECOMMENDATIONS

Though some risk factors for developing prostate cancer are not modifiable, several are. As with some other cancers, a higher body mass index (BMI) is an independent risk factor for prostate cancer. Although increased risk from higher BMI seems greatest among African American men, a higher BMI among non-Hispanic white men also increases risk for development of prostate cancer and even of higher grade prostate cancer. African American men with a BMI greater than 35 had a 4 times higher rate of developing prostate cancer than those with BMI less than 25. A mechanism for this association is unknown; however, lowering a patient's BMI could lower the risk of prostate cancer.[17]

Table 1
Estimated effects after 13 years of inviting men aged 55 to 69 years in the United States to prostate-specific antigen–based screening for prostate cancer (current as of May 2018)[a]

Group Description	Number of Men Affected
Men invited to screening	1000
Men who received at least 1 positive PSA test result	240
Men who have undergone 1 or more transrectal prostate biopsies	220[b]
Men hospitalized for a biopsy complication	2
Men diagnosed with prostate cancer	100
Men who initially received active treatment with radical prostatectomy or radiation therapy	65
Men who initially received active surveillance	30
Men who initially received active surveillance who went on to receive active treatment with radical prostatectomy or radiation therapy	15
Men with sexual dysfunction who received initial or deferred treatment	50
Men with urinary incontinence who received initial or deferred treatment	15
Men who avoided metastatic prostate cancer	3
Men who died of causes other than prostate cancer	200
Men who died of prostate cancer despite screening, diagnosis, and treatment	5
Men who avoided dying of prostate cancer	1.3

Abbreviations: PIVOT, Prostate Cancer Intervention versus Observation Trial; ProtecT, Prostate Testing for Cancer and Treatment; SPCG-4=Scandinavian Prostate Cancer Group Study Number 4
[a] Estimates based on benefits observed in the European Randomized Study of Screening for Prostate Cancer (ERSPC) trial for men aged 55 to 69 years and on treatment harms derived from pooled absolute rates in the treatment groups in the 3 treatment trials (ProtecT, PIVOT, SPCG-4).
[b] Result based on biopsy rate in the ERSPC trial. Current practice in the United States will likely result in fewer biopsies. The potential effect of fewer biopsies on other outcomes, including reductions in prostate cancer diagnosis and mortality, are not clear.
From U.S. Preventive Services Task Force. Final recommendation statement: prostate cancer: screening. Rockville, MD. May 2018. Available at: https://www.uspreventiveservicestaskforce.org/Page/Document/RecommendationStatementFinal/prostate-cancer-screening1. Accessed September 06, 2018; Used with permission of the U.S. Preventive Services Task Force.

The role of 5-alpha-reductase inhibitors in prevention have also generated much attention. Original investigations suggested that there might be a decrease in prostate cancer diagnosis but an increased likelihood of developing advanced malignancy. Two randomized controlled trials, the Prostate Cancer Prevention Trial[18] and the Reduction by Dutasteride of Prostate Cancer Events,[19] showed risk reduction greater than 20% but increased risk of diagnosis with high-grade prostate cancer compared with placebo. Recent studies have downplayed this risk, offering some reassurance; however, large-scale studies are still needed given the use of this class of medicine for benign prostatic hypertrophy relief.[20] The US Food and Drug Administration currently warns against the use of 5-alpha-reductase inhibitors for chemoprevention of prostate cancer.

A large randomized controlled trial followed men without prostate cancer for between 7 and 12 years and found that vitamin E supplementation (400 IU/d) led to a statistically significant increase in prostate cancer. Biological explanations for this association are still a mystery; however, investigators caution against common over-the-counter supplementation with vitamin E and risks related to developing prostate cancer. Taking vitamin E and selenium together did not increase risk.[21]

The lack of robust preventative data has led to an overall lack of preventative recommendations, which can meaningfully affect patient care. Combined with screening recommendations previously outlined, prostate cancer prevention will continue to be an area warranting further exploration.

Soy-based foods and isoflavones do seem to decrease risk. One review found that the decrease in risk was significant only for total soy intake or nonfermented soy foods. The studies reviewed, however, varied in populations studied, with different outcomes for different populations. This decreased cancer risk was only significant for studies conducted of Asian populations, not Western populations.[22] Another review combined 2 studies of soy isoflavones, with a total of 122 men, and reported a risk ratio of 0.49 (95% CI 0.26–0.95).

A high intake of cruciferous vegetables reduces the risk of prostate cancer.[23] Other dietary patterns have less convincing evidence. The literature on coffee consumption provides variable results. Fish intake may decrease the risk of prostate cancer-based mortality.

Vitamin E or selenium supplementation does not seem to prevent prostate cancer.[24] Though study findings differ, low-dose multiple antioxidant vitamin supplementation may reduce the risk.[25] Aspirin and other nonsteroidal antiinflammatory drugs use may reduce risk of prostate cancer.[26]

Vasectomy does not increase risk.[27] High ejaculation frequency associated with decreased risk of prostate cancer. Compared with men who ejaculated 4 to 7 times per month during a period of their lives, men who ejaculated more than 20 times per month had an adjusted relative risk of 0.67 (95% CI 0.51–0.89) for prostate cancer.[28] However, men with the lowest ejaculation frequency also had a reduced association with prostate cancer.[29]

OUTCOMES FOR PATIENTS AND COMPLICATIONS

Commonly used therapies in the past included prostatectomy, EBRT, and brachytherapy. Although much of the controversy related to prostate cancer has centered on screening, the treatments are also controversial because of the estimated risks and benefits to patients. Treatment is controversial because most elderly men will have prostate cancer noted incidentally at autopsy, and treatment can cause significant adverse effects.

To guide therapy, the Gleason score helps to identify prostate cancer that merits more or less aggressive therapeutic approaches. Using the current standard of 10 to 12 biopsy specimens, and scoring the most prevalent and second most prevalent histopathologic patterns on a scale of 1 to 5, with 5 being the highest risk, the Gleason score ranges from 2 to 10. A Gleason score of 6 or below is considered lowest risk, 7 is intermediate, and 8 or above is high risk.

Given the risk of adverse effects from other treatment approaches, active surveillance represents a viable option for men newly diagnosed with low-average risk of aggressive disease. This approach includes regular PSA testing, DRE, and possibly MRI. Also, if indicated, repeat prostate biopsy is done at 6 to 12 month intervals before curative treatment is attempted.[30] In a randomized controlled trial following more than 8000 British men, active surveillance was compared with radical prostatectomy or radiation therapy for men with localized prostate cancer. After 10 years, 3 out of 100 men were more likely to have metastatic disease. The percentage of men followed over

10 years who had pursued curative approaches increased over time; however, half of men avoided aggressive therapy without impact on disease-specific or all-cause mortality.[31]

Another study compared radical prostatectomy, ERBT, and active surveillance, and the symptoms associated with each approach. Men undergoing radical prostatectomy were more likely to have sexual dysfunction and urinary incontinence compared with ERBT or surveillance. Men in the active surveillance cohort were more likely to develop urinary irritative symptoms.[8]

Chen and colleagues[9] compared active surveillance, ERBT, brachytherapy, and radical prostatectomy with active surveillance, monitoring short-term symptoms with those at 24 months. Again, surgery was associated with more sexual and pathologic incontinence. ERBT and brachytherapy were associated with urinary irritation and obstruction, and ERBT with bowel symptoms. However, at 24 months, no significant differences existed between groups.

REFERENCES

1. Barry MJ. Screening for prostate cancer—the controversy that refuses to die [Editorial]. N Engl J Med 2009;360:1351–4.
2. Vickers AJ. Prostate cancer screening: time to question how to optimize the ratio of benefits and harms. Ann Intern Med 2017;167(7):509–10.
3. Litwin MS, Tan HJ. The diagnosis and treatment of prostate cancer: a review. JAMA 2017;317(24):2532–42.
4. Mulhem E, Fulbright N, Duncan N. Prostate cancer screening. Am Fam Physician 2015;92(8):683–8.
5. Hoffman RM. Clinical practice. Screening for prostate cancer. N Engl J Med 2011; 365(21):2013–9.
6. Pinsky PF, Prorok PC, Kramer BJ. Prostate cancer screening. N Engl J Med 2017; 376(24):2402.
7. Barry MJ, Hayes JH. Evaluating an elevated screening PSA test. JAMA 2015; 314(19):2073–4.
8. Barocas DA, Alvarez J, Resnick MJ, et al. Association between radiation therapy, surgery, or observation for localized prostate cancer and patient-reported outcomes after 3 years. JAMA 2017;317(11):1126–40.
9. Chen RC, Basak R, Meyer AM, et al. Association between choice of radical prostatectomy, external beam radiotherapy, brachytherapy, or active surveillance and patient-reported quality of life among men with localized prostate cancer. JAMA 2017;317(11):1141–50.
10. Haas GP, Delongchamps N, Brawley OW, et al. The worldwide epidemiology of prostate cancer: perspectives from autopsy studies. Can J Urol 2008;15(1): 3866–71.
11. Jahn JL, Giovannucci EL, Stampfer MJ. The high prevalence of undiagnosed prostate cancer at autopsy: implications for epidemiology and treatment of prostate cancer in the prostate-specific antigen-era. Int J Cancer 2015;137(12): 2795–802.
12. Hemminki K. Familial risk and familial survival in prostate cancer. World J Urol 2012;30(2):143–8.
13. Odedina FT, Akinremi TO, Chinegwundoh F, et al. Prostate cancer disparities in Black men of African descent: a comparative literature review of prostate cancer burden among Black men in the United States, Caribbean, United Kingdom, and West Africa. Infect Agent Cancer 2009;4(Suppl 1):S2.

14. US Preventive Services Task Force. Screening for prostate cancer: US preventive services task force recommendation statement. JAMA 2018;319(18):1901–13.
15. Ilic D, Neuberger MM, Djulbegovic M, et al. Screening for prostate cancer. Cochrane Database Syst Rev 2013;(1):CD004720.
16. Schröder FH, Hugosson J, Roobol MJ, et al. The European randomized study of screening for prostate cancer – prostate cancer mortality at 13 years of follow-up. Lancet 2014;384(9959):2027–35.
17. Thomas CR Jr. Targeted reduction in body mass index is a worthwhile risk reduction strategy for prostate cancer. JAMA Oncol 2015;1(3):349.
18. Lucia MS, Epstein JI, Goodman PJ, et al. Finasteride and high-grade prostate cancer in the prostate cancer prevention trial. J Natl Cancer Inst 2007;99(18):1375–83.
19. Andriole GL, Bostwick DG, Brawley OW, et al, REDUCE Study Group. Effect of dutasteride on the risk of prostate cancer. N Engl J Med 2010;362(13):1192–202.
20. Azoulay L, Eberg M, Benayoun S, et al. 5α-reductase inhibitors and the risk of cancer-related mortality in men with prostate cancer. JAMA Oncol 2015;1(3):314–20.
21. Klein EA, Thompson IM Jr, Tangen CM, et al. Vitamin E and the risk of prostate cancer: the selenium and Vitamin E cancer prevention trial (SELECT). JAMA 2011;306(14):1549–56.
22. Yan L, Spitznagel E. Soy consumption and prostate cancer risk in med: a revisit of a meta-analysis. Am J Clin Nutr 2009;4:1155–63.
23. Kirsh VA, Peters U, Mayne ST, et al. Prostate, lung, colorectal and ovarian cancer screening trial. Prospective study of fruit and vegetable intake and risk of prostate cancer. J Natl Cancer Inst 2007;99:1200–9.
24. Lippman SM, Klein EA, Goodman PJ, et al. Effect of selenium and vitamin E on risk of prostate cancer and other cancers: the Selenium and Vitamin E Cancer Prevention Trial (SELECT). JAMA 2009;301(1):39–51.
25. Hercberg S, Galan P, Preziosi P, et al. The SU.VI.MAX Study: a randomized, placebo-controlled trial of the health effects of antioxidant vitamins and minerals. Arch Intern Med 2004;164(21):2335–42 [Erratum: Arch Intern Med. 2005;165(3):286].
26. Vidal AC, Howard LE, Moreira DM, et al. Aspirin, NSAIDs, and risk of prostate cancer: results from the REDUCE study. Clin Cancer Res 2015;21(4):756–62.
27. Nayan M, Hamilton RJ, Macdonald EM, et al, Canadian Drug Safety and Effectiveness Research Network(CDSERN). Vasectomy and risk of prostate cancer: population based matched cohort study. BMJ 2016;355:i5546.
28. Leitzmann MF, Platz EA, Stampfer MJ, et al. Ejaculation frequency and subsequent risk of prostate cancer. JAMA 2004;291(13):1578–86.
29. Wellbery C. Frequency of ejaculation and risk for prostate cancer. Am Fam Physician 2005;71(2):369–70.
30. Matulewicz RS, Weiner AB, Schaeffer EM. Active surveillance for prostate cancer. JAMA 2017;318(21):2152.
31. Ebell M. Active surveillance of localized prostate cancer: no increased mortality, but higher rate of clinical progression. AFP 2017;95(3):196.

Screening for Sexually Transmitted Diseases

Shoshana B. Levy, MD, MPH*, Jyothi Gunta, MD, MPH[1],
Peter Edemekong, MD, MPH

KEYWORDS

- Sexually transmitted disease screening • Sexually transmitted infection screening
- Chlamydia • Gonorrhea • Syphilis • HIV

KEY POINTS

- By screening the appropriate populations for sexually transmitted infections (STIs), we can treat affected individuals (secondary prevention), prevent fetal abnormalities (primary prevention), and prevent spread of the infection to others (primary prevention).
- Screening for chlamydia and gonorrhea should be offered to all sexually active women under the age of 25, pregnant women, men who have sex with men (MSM), and those with HIV.
- Syphilis screening should be offered to pregnant women, MSM, and those with human immunodeficiency virus (HIV). Nonpregnant women and heterosexual men should be screened if they are at elevated risk.
- HIV screening should be performed at least once on all sexually active individuals. Pregnant women should be screened with every pregnancy and MSM should be screened annually.
- Do not screen for herpes simplex virus in asymptomatic individuals.

INTRODUCTION

Sexually transmitted infections (STIs) remain prevalent in our society despite decades of prevention and treatment campaigns. The Centers for Disease Control and Prevention (CDC) estimates that the annual incidence of all STIs in the United States is 20 million and the prevalence is 110 million.[1] Half of new infections occur in those under the age of 25. The most common STIs in the United States in order of incidence are HPV (human papillomavirus), chlamydia, trichomoniasis, gonorrhea, genital herpes, syphilis, human

Disclosure Statement: The authors have nothing to disclose.
Residency in General Preventive Medicine and Public Health, Florida Department of Health, Palm Beach County, 800 Clematis, West Palm Beach, FL 33401, USA
[1] Present address: 2392 Wrotham Terrace, Wellington, FL 33414.
* Corresponding author.
E-mail address: Shoshana.levy@flhealth.gov

Prim Care Clin Office Pract 46 (2019) 157–173
https://doi.org/10.1016/j.pop.2018.10.013
0095-4543/19/© 2018 Elsevier Inc. All rights reserved.

immunodeficiency virus (HIV), and hepatitis B.[1] In 2016, there were more than 2 million cases of diagnosed chlamydia, gonorrhea, and syphilis infections alone.[2]

In 2010, it was estimated that STIs cost the US economy $16 billion per year in both direct and indirect costs.[1] Many of these diseases can be asymptomatic or the symptoms may be mistaken for other more benign conditions.[2] Asymptomatic individuals can unknowingly transmit infections to their sexual partners.[2] The sequelae of the various STIs can be serious and include infertility, pelvic inflammatory disorder, fetal abnormalities, cancer, and death.[2]

Screening of asymptomatic individuals is important to the control of STIs in the US population. We as providers need to improve our screening efforts. Insurance data from 2014 show that 47% of sexually active women under the age of 24 with commercial health insurance and 54.6% with Medicaid were screened for chlamydia.[3] By screening the appropriate populations, we can treat affected individuals (secondary prevention), prevent fetal abnormalities (primary prevention), and prevent spread of the infection to others (primary prevention).[2]

In order to know who to screen, providers must determine risk factors by taking a sexual history. It is important to ask about risk factors in a nonjudgmental manner. The CDC has published a guide and a mnemonic for taking a sexual history called the Five Ps, which are as follows[4,5]:

- *P*ast history of sexually transmitted diseases (STDs):
  - "Have you ever had an STD in the past?"[4]
- *P*artners:
  - "Have you had sex with men, women, or both?[4]
  - "In the past 6 months, how many people have you had sex with?"[4]
  - "Have any of your sex partners in the past 12 months had sex with other partners while they were still in a sexual relationship with you?"[4]
- *P*ractices:
  - "Do you have vaginal sex, anal sex, and/or oral sex?"[4]
  - "Have you ever used needles to inject/shoot drugs?"[4]
- *P*rotection from STDs:
  - "What do you do to prevent STDs and HIV?"[4]
  - "Tell me about your use of condoms with your recent partner."[4]
- *P*revention of Pregnancy:
  - "How would it be for you if you were to get pregnant now?"[4]
  - "What are you doing to prevent pregnancy?"[4]

In this article, the authors have chosen to focus on reportable STIs, which include gonorrhea, chlamydia, syphilis, and HIV, as well as brief recommendations for hepatitis B and C, trichomonas, and genital herpes screening. The authors have summarized the recommendations from various organizations that produce screening recommendations (eg, US Preventive Services Task Force [USPSTF], Centers for Disease Control and Prevention [CDC], American College of Obstetricians and Gynecologists (ACOG), American Academy of Family Physicians (AAF), and American Academy of Pediatrics [AAP]). All patients diagnosed with infections should abstain from sexual activity until infection is resolved and they and partners finish treatment. Remember these recommendations only apply to asymptomatic individuals.[6] Once an individual has symptoms, testing is diagnostic, which is beyond the scope of this review.

It is important to know the prevalence in your population. If you work in a population with a high prevalence of a specific disease or that has particular risky sexual practices, consider screening regardless of recommendations.[6]

CHLAMYDIA TRACHOMATIS AND *NEISSERIA GONORRHOEAE*
Introduction

Chlamydia trachomatis and *Neisseria gonorrhoeae* are the most commonly reported STIs in the United States.[2] In 2016, there were 468,514 cases of gonorrhea (145.8 cases per 100,000 people) and 1,598,354 cases of chlamydia (497.3 cases per 100,000 people).[4] It is difficult to know the true incidence of gonorrhea and chlamydia because many infections are asymptomatic. According to the CDC, there are more than 800,000 persons infected with gonorrhea in the United States each year, but only half of these infections are diagnosed and reported.[7]

Untreated chlamydia and gonorrhea in women can lead to serious complications, such as pelvic inflammatory disease (PID), infertility, neonatal complications, and chronic pelvic pain.[6] Forty-six percent of new infections occur in women aged 15 to 24.[7] Screening for gonorrhea and chlamydia reduces complications in women who are at increased risk for these diseases.[6]

The USPSTF concluded that there is not enough evidence to determine whether there is a net benefit to screen all men (grade I).[8] However, men who have sex with men (MSM) are at a high risk for chlamydia and gonorrhea. Higher frequency of unsafe sexual practices, multiple sex partners, and substance use place MSM at increased risk for STIs.[6]

Table 1 summarizes the USPSTF recommendations for chlamydia and gonorrhea screening, and **Table 2** provides additional risk factors to consider in screening decisions.

Special Populations and Screening

The CDC recommends screening women aged 35 and younger upon intake in juvenile detention or jail facilities.[9] They also recommend retesting pregnant women in the third trimester if they have continued risk for infection and in those who test positive at their first prenatal visit.[9]

There have been several trials that suggest that screening young women for chlamydia and gonorrhea reduces the rate of PID. One large randomized controlled trial found that screening and treating women at increased risk for chlamydia was associated with reduced incidence of PID (relative risk, 0.44 [95% confidence interval, 0.20–0.90]).[15] Another study of women in London found that of women who tested positive for chlamydia at baseline, there was a decreased incidence of PID and that most episodes of PID occurred in women who had tested negative at baseline and subsequently tested positive.[6] These findings support the need for repeated screening over time to prevent ongoing chlamydial transmission among at-risk individuals.

The AAP recommends screening adolescents and young adults exposed to chlamydia or gonorrhea in the past 60 days. They also recommend annual screening for chlamydia in sexually active men in high prevalence settings, such as jail or juvenile correction facilities; national job training programs; STI clinics; high school clinics; and adolescent clinics.[11]

Most men with *C trachomatis* and *N gonorrhoeae* present with symptoms. Men with these infections will present with urethritis and epididymitis, prompting timely treatment and prevention of complications.[6] There is no clear additional benefit to screen men who have sex with women only.[8] It is reasonable to screen heterosexual men for chlamydia in high prevalence settings, such as at adolescent clinics and correctional facilities. Screening is more relevant among MSM, because they have a high burden of STIs. The MSM population should be screened at least annually regardless of condom use and more if assessed to be at increased risk.[9]

Table 1
Screening for chlamydia and gonorrhea: summary of recommendations*

Gender	Population	Recommendation	Screening Frequency	Comments
Women	Sexually active <25 y	Screen for chlamydia and gonorrhea	Annually[a]	Screen more frequently for those at increased risk (see **Table 2**)
	Sexually active ≥25 y	No routine screening		Targeted CT/GC screening for women with risk factors (see **Table 2**)
	HIV positive	Screen all HIV positive women up to 64 y of age	Annually	Repeat according to level of risk (see **Table 2**)
	Pregnant	Screen all pregnant women (vaginal, cervical, or urine)	First trimester	Repeat screening in third trimester if at increased risk (see **Table 2**)
Men	Heterosexual men	No recommended routine screening		Targeted screening for CT in high-risk settings (see **Table 2**)
	MSM	CT and GC (urine)	Annually	Repeat screening every 3–6 mo, as indicated by risk
		CT and GC (rectal)	Annually (if exposed)	
		GC (pharyngeal)	Annually (if exposed)	
	HIV positive	CT and GC (urine)	Annually	Repeat screening every 3–6 mo, as indicated by risk.
		CT and GC (rectal)	Annually (if exposed)	
		GC (pharyngeal)	Annually (if exposed)	

Abbreviations: CT, chlamydia; GC, gonorrhea.
[a] Although USPSTF did not find any evidence to suggest specific screening frequencies, CDC and others recommend annual screening in this population.
Data from Refs.[8–12]

Table 2
Risk factors for gonorrhea, chlamydia, and syphilis by population

Population	Risk Factors
Women	• Prior CT or GC infection, particularly in the past 24 mo • >1 sex partner in the past year • Partner with concurrent partners • New partner in the past 3 mo • Partner with STI • Transactional sex (eg, drugs, money, housing) • Inconsistent condom use and not in mutually monogamous relationship • Intravenous (IV) drug users and/or partners who are IV drug users • High-prevalence population, such as incarcerated, military recruit, public STI clinic
MSM	• Multiple or anonymous partners • IV drugs use • Sex in conjunction with illicit drug use, including methamphetamine • Receptive or insertive anal sex • Oral sex with partners who have syphilis sores or lesions • Partners who engage in the above activities

Men who have sex with women	• Prior infection (in past 24 mo)
	• IV drug use
	• High-risk setting such as
	  ○ Adolescent clinics
	  ○ Correctional facilities
	  ○ STD clinics
	  ○ National job training programs

Data from Refs.[8–14]

Screening Tests

Nucleic acid amplification tests

Nucleic acid amplification test (NAAT) is the gold standard for screening/testing for gonorrhea and chlamydia because it yields the best sensitivity and specificity. NAAT can be used on specimens collected from first-catch urine or self-collected vaginal swabs.[12] For women undergoing a speculum examination, or for high-risk women undergoing routine Pap smear, NAAT can be performed on endocervical or vaginal swabs.[9] Rectal and pharyngeal swabs should be collected from persons who engage in receptive anal intercourse and oral sex. The Food and Drug Administration has not approved NAAT for testing these specimens.[11] The sensitivity and specificity of urine specimens in women are equal to those from the endocervix, vagina, and male urethra. The same specimen is used to test for both chlamydia and gonorrhea.[11]

Culture

Cultures are not routinely used in clinical practice, because they are expensive and require technical expertise. Cultures are used for chlamydia research and reference laboratories.[9] Cultures are used to assess antibiotic susceptibilities in gonorrhea. Cultures are still important due to gonococcal resistance to several classes of antibiotics.[9]

Serology

C trachomatis serology (complement fixation titers >1:64) can be used to diagnose chlamydia. There is a lack of standardization. Serology requires high levels of expertise to interpret. It does not diagnose rectal infections in men and it does diagnose upper genital tract infection in women.[9]

Antigen detection
The antigen detection method is invasive, requiring a swab from the cervix or urethra.[9] It is only useful when there is a high prevalence of infection.

Genetic probe methods
The genetic probe method is invasive, requiring usage of a direct swab from the cervix or urethra. The sensitivity is considerably lower than NAAT and is not used frequently.[9]

Gram stain
Gram stain is used for diagnosis of gonorrhea urethritis in a symptomatic man. This test is highly specific.[9]

Treatment

The CDC releases updated guidelines for the treatment of STDs every few years as well as guidelines for offering expedited partner therapy. **Table 3** is a summary of the CDC's 2015 treatment guidelines.

Table 3
Centers for Disease Control and Prevention: updated recommended treatment regimens for gonococcal and chlamydial infections

Disease		
Gonorrhea	First-line treatment	• Ceftriaxone 250 mg in a single intramuscular dose + Azithromycin 1 g orally in a single dose or doxycycline 100 mg orally bid for 7 d[a]
	Alternative regimens	• Cefixime 400 mg in a single oral dose + Azithromycin 1 g orally in a single dose or doxycycline 100 mg orally bid for 7 d[a] + Test of cure in 1 wk If the patient has severe cephalosporin allergy: • Azithromycin 2 g in a single oral dose + Gemifloxacin 320 mg in a single oral dose + Test of cure in 1 wk
	Uncomplicated gonococcal infections of the pharynx: first-line treatment	• Ceftriaxone 250 mg in a single intramuscular dose + Azithromycin 1 g orally in a single dose or doxycycline 100 mg orally bid for 7 d[a]
Chlamydia	First-line treatment	• Azithromycin 1 g orally in a single dose • Doxycycline 100 mg orally twice a day for 7 d
	Alternative regimens	• Erythromycin base 500 mg orally 4 times a day for 7 d • Erythromycin ethylsuccinate 800 mg orally 4 times a day for 7 d • Levofloxacin 500 mg orally once daily for 7 d • Ofloxacin 300 mg orally twice a day for 7 d

[a] Because of resistance, only use alternatives if the patient is highly allergic to azithromycin.
    Data from Centers for Disease Control and Prevention. 2015 sexually transmitted diseases treatment guidelines. Available at: https://www.cdc.gov/std/tg2015/gonorrhea.htm. Accessed March 28, 2018; and Chlamydial infections. Centers for Disease Control and Prevention; 2015. Available at: https://www.cdc.gov/std/tg2015/chlamydia.htm. Accessed March 28, 2018.

Sexual contacts of positive cases should be notified, examined, and treated for identified or suspected STD. In some settings, expedited partner therapy can be used in order to prevent spread of disease.[16]

SYPHILIS
Introduction

After a decline in the early 2000s, syphilis (*Treponema pallidum*) has been making a comeback. There were 27,814 reported cases of syphilis in 2016 at a rate of 9/100,000 people.[17] MSM between the ages of 20 and 29 accounted for most cases in 2014.[18]

Syphilis is spread by direct contact with a sore during vaginal, anal, or oral sex. The infection is divided into primary, secondary, latent, and tertiary stages. Early stage disease can be mild and not noticed. Primary syphilis often presents as one or multiple sores at the original site of infection. Secondary syphilis presents as rash, swollen lymph nodes, and fever. Latent syphilis has no signs or symptoms. Tertiary syphilis occurs years to decades after initial infection and results in end organ damage in the brain, heart, and other major organs.[17] Congenital syphilis can result in severe sequelae, such as miscarriage, stillbirth, death shortly after birth, blindness, deafness, hepatosplenomegaly, and pseudo-paralysis.[19–21]

USPSTF recommends that pregnant women as well as certain high-risk groups be screened. **Table 4** provides screening recommendations.

Special Populations and Screening

The prevalence of congenital syphilis in the general population is low.[17] However, because congenital syphilis is so devastating, all pregnant women should be screened for syphilis regardless of risk factors.[22] The number of congenital syphilis cases has gone up in recent years from a low of 8.4/100,000 live births in 2012 to a rate of 15.7/100,000 live births in 2016.[2] In higher-risk populations, women should be screened in the third trimester as well.[9]

Table 4				
Screening for syphilis: summary of recommendations				
Gender	**Population**	**Recommendation**	**Screening Frequency**	**Comments**
Women	Pregnant women	Screen at first prenatal visit	Every pregnancy	Use RPR. Retest early in the third trimester and at delivery if at high risk (see **Table 2**)
	Sexually active	No routine screening		Targeted screening for women with risk factors (see **Table 2**)
	HIV positive	Screen all women up to age 64	Annually	May screen more often depending on risk factors
Men	Heterosexual men	No routine screening		Targeted screening in high-risk settings or risk factors (see **Table 2**)
	MSM	Screen if sexually active	Annually	Repeat screening every 3 mo, as indicated by risk
	HIV positive	Screen	Annually	Repeat screening every 3 mo, as indicated by risk

Data from Refs.[13,21,24]

The burden of syphilis in MSM is higher than in any other groups. Eighty-nine percent of syphilis cases in 2016 were in men, and 81% of those were in MSM.[17] For MSM living with HIV, syphilis infection increases HIV viral load and decreases CD4 cell counts.[23] Syphilis also increases the risk for HIV infection.[23] Approximately one-half of MSM diagnosed with syphilis are coinfected with HIV.[17]

Providers should be aware of syphilis prevalence in their community when deciding whom to screen. There is a higher prevalence of syphilis in men who are incarcerated, men who have a history of commercial sex work, certain racial/ethnic groups, or those younger than 29.[13]

Screening and Confirmation Tests

For screening nontreponemal tests should be used
There are 2 main types of tiers used for screening: Venereal Disease Research Laboratory and Rapid Plasma Regain (RPR). Titers reduce with adequate therapy.[24] Both tests have a sensitivity of 44% to 77% depending on stage with a specificity of 85%.[25–27]

Confirmation Confirmatory testing is performed by treponemal-specific serology. All serology testing remains positive for life once someone has been infected.

There are several different serology tests. The most often used tests are *T pallidum* hemagglutination and *T pallidum* particle agglutination due to their high sensitivity and specificity.[28–30] Fluorescent treponemal antibody absorbed test is used less often due to lower specificity.[28]

Definite confirmation Definite confirmation is done with Darkfield microscopy. It requires a skin/lesion biopsy, which would not be available when screening asymptomatic individuals.[28]

Treatment
Uncomplicated syphilis should be treated with parenteral penicillin G benzathine (**Table 5**). Treatment should be dispensed on site.[31] All sex partners from the previous 60 days should be evaluated. The patient should be abstinent until they and their partners are treated.[4] Pregnant women should be treated immediately. If the woman has a penicillin allergy, desensitize to penicillin and treat to reduce the risk of congenital syphilis.[24]

Partner notification As with chlamydia and gonorrhea, this is a reportable disease, and a contact investigation should be performed by the proper authorities and all contacts treated.

HUMAN IMMUNODEFICIENCY VIRUS
Introduction

HIV is the virus that leads to AIDS. Since its emergence in the 1980s, HIV infection has transitioned from a death sentence due to opportunistic infections, to a chronic disease. There is no cure for HIV, but treatment helps control the infection and enables persons with HIV to live a long life.[33] About 40,000 people a year become infected with HIV in the United States, and an estimated 1.1 million people are living with HIV in the United States.[33] About 1 out of 7 persons living with HIV does not know they are infected.[33] HIV remains a major global public health issue.[34]

The symptoms of HIV vary depending on the stage of the infection. Individuals infected with HIV are often unaware of their infection in the first few months after

Table 5		
Centers for Disease Control and Prevention recommended treatment regimens for syphilis infections		
	Stage	

Primary, secondary, or early latent syphilis (<1 y)	• Benzathine penicillin G 2.4 million units IM in a single dose
	• If allergic to penicillin:
	  ○ Doxycycline 100 mg PO BID × 14 d
	  ○ Tetracycline 500 mg PO four times daily × 14 d	

Late latent (>1 y), latent syphilis of unknown duration or tertiary syphilis with normal cerebrospinal fluid examination	Benzathine penicillin G 2.4 million units IM × 3 doses at 1-wk intervals If allergic to penicillin: Doxycycline 100 mg PO BID × 28 d tetracycline 500 mg po four times daily × 28 d	
Pregnant women	Treat with appropriate penicillin regimen for stage of infection. Additional doses may be indicted if evidence of fetal syphilis on ultrasound	
Syphilis patients with HIV infection	No additional doses of benzathine penicillin are indicated	

Abbreviations: IM, intramuscularly; PO, orally.
Data from Refs.[24,31,32]

contracting the virus, when they are the most infectious.[33] In the first few weeks after infection, individuals may be completely asymptomatic or may experience a mild flu-like illness.[35] If left untreated, the virus attacks the T cells or CD4 cells, which fight infections, thereby increasing the risk of progression to AIDS.[35]

Early identification and treatment of HIV-infected persons are associated with reduced risk for progression to AIDS and AIDS-related events and death.[35] Early identification and treatment of HIV-positive pregnant women significantly reduce the risk of transmission from mother to child.[36]

Table 6 summarizes screening recommendations for HIV.

Special Populations and Screening

There is a higher proportion of MSM living with HIV than any other group in the United States.[37] About 1 in 6 MSM living with HIV is unaware of their infection. Anal sex carries the most risk of contracting or transferring HIV.[37] High-risk individuals should have a repeat HIV testing at least once a year.[41] For asymptomatic MSM, routine and frequent screening should be considered based on individual risk factors, local epidemiology, and local policies. In addition, providers should screen patients for appropriateness for preexposure prophylaxis (PrEP).[42] PrEP is prescribed for individuals engaging in high-risk behavior making them susceptible to HIV infection including members of discordant couples where one partner is HIV positive and one is not.[42]

Screening pregnant women for HIV infection is important because treatment of the mother greatly reduces the risk of transmission to the infant.[34] If status is unknown or cannot be confirmed at time of delivery, screen before discharge with a rapid test.[38] HIV can be transmitted through many bodily fluids, including breastmilk.[40] HIV-positive women should not breastfeed their children. Initiation of antiretroviral therapy in pregnant women has kept the rate of perinatal HIV transmission at less than 1% in the United States.[40]

Table 6
Screening for human immunodeficiency virus: summary of recommendations

Gender	Population	Recommendation	Screening Frequency	Comments
Women	Nonpregnant sexually active 13–65 years old	One-time screening	Once	Consider screening more frequently if at increased risk (see **Table 2**)[a]
	Pregnant women	Screen at first prenatal visit	Every pregnancy	Repeat testing in the third trimester if increased risk of HIV
Men	Sexually active heterosexual men 13–65 years old	One-time screen	Once	Consider screening more frequently if at increased risk
	MSM	Screen	Annually (if sexually active)	Screen more often if more than one partner since most recent HIV testing

[a] HIV is more prevalent in the southern states, minorities (African Americans and Hispanic/Latinos) as well as transgender individuals.
Data from Refs.[36–40]

Human Immunodeficiency Virus: Preferred and Gold Standard Screening and Confirmatory Test

Screening

HIV screening uses a fourth-generation antigen/antibody combination HIV-1/2 immunoassay plus a confirmatory HIV-1/HIV-2 antibody differentiation immunoassay.[43] The criteria for a positive HIV test include a positive combination assay or enzyme-linked immunosorbent assay (ELISA) followed by a positive confirmatory assay.[43] A negative test is a negative screening combination assay or ELISA. An intermediate result is when the combination assay or ELISA is positive but the confirmatory test is intermediate or negative.[43]

Antibody-only tests ELISA is a third-generation antibody test that detects immunoglobulin M (IgM) and IgG antibodies to HIV as early as 3 weeks after the infection.[44]

Combination human immunodeficiency virus antigen and antibody tests Combination human immunodeficiency virus antigen and antibody test is a fourth-generation test that can detect HIV p24 antigen in addition to both antibodies to HIV-1 and HIV-2.[44]

Confirmatory tests

Human immunodeficiency virus-1/human immunodeficiency virus-2 differentiation immunoassay HIV-1/HIV-2 differentiation immunoassay is a rapid test used to confirm positive fourth-generation combination assay and to distinguish between HIV-1 and HIV-2 infection.[43]

Western blot Western blot test is used to confirm a positive ELISA test. This test can detect IgG antibody to HIV-1 and a special western blot must be requested to detect HIV-2 antibody.[44]

Viral detection Viral detection test can be used to establish HIV diagnosis because virus is present in blood samples before HIV antibodies can be detected. The most common methods used detect HIV RNA or HIV p24 antigen.[44]

Rapid diagnostic tests Rapid diagnostic tests offer same-day results with an opportunity to discuss care and treatment options before the patient leaves the clinic.

Treatment

The most effective treatments include the use of combined highly active antiretroviral therapy (3 or more antiretroviral agents administered together, usually from 2 or more classes), immunizations, and prophylaxis for opportunistic infections.[35] Further details on treatment of HIV are beyond the scope of this article.

HEPATITIS B AND C
Introduction

Hepatitis is a generic term for any disease that causes inflammation of the liver. Hepatitis can be either self-limiting or can progress to fibrosis, cirrhosis, or liver cancer.[45] There are 5 main viruses that cause hepatitis: A, B, C, D, and E. Hepatitis B and C can be sexually transmitted and are the most common viral causes of liver cirrhosis and cancer.[45]

Hepatitis B

About 21,000 Americans are infected with hepatitis B every year, and there are about 2.2 million people in the United States with chronic hepatitis B.[46] The highest percentage of infections comes from foreign born individuals from Asia, Pacific Islands, and Africa.[46] Hepatitis B is transmitted through direct contact with infected blood, semen, or another body fluid which can happen during sexual contact, needle sticks, and birth from mother to child.[47] Risk for chronic infection is directly correlated with age at infection. About 90% of infected infants will develop chronic infections, whereas only 2% to 6% of infected adults will.[47] The hepatitis B vaccine is very effective and has substantially decreased the prevalence of chronic hepatitis B in the native-born population.[46]

Hepatitis C

About 41,000 Americans are infected with hepatitis C every year.[46] The United States has more than 3 million people living with chronic hepatitis C; however, that number has likely decreased due to recent effective treatments that have come on the market.[46] Seventy-five percent to 85% of those infected will develop chronic infection.[46] Cirrhosis due to chronic hepatitis C is the leading indication for liver transplantation in the United States.[48] The most common route of transmission is through needles and syringe sharing by injection drug users, but it can also be transmitted through sexual contact with an infected partner.[46] There is no vaccine for hepatitis C.

Tables 7 and **8** summarize the risk factors that increase the transmission of hepatitis B and C.

Screening Methods for Hepatitis B

There are several different serologic tests that are used in order to determine immune status. For most screening, hepatitis B surface antigen (HbsAg) is sufficient. HbsAg will be negative if the patient is not infected and positive if they are. In order to find immune status as well, the hepatitis B surface antibody (anti-HBs) and the hepatitis B core antibody (anti-HBc) should be tested. **Table 9** provides interpretation of these results.

Screening Methods for Hepatitis C

To screen, an HCV antibody test should be used. If positive, a confirmatory HCV RNA test should be ordered.

Table 7
Screening recommendations for hepatitis B and hepatitis C

Virus	Population	Recommendation	Frequency	Notes
Hepatitis B	Women	Screen if at increased risk	No recommended intervals	See **Table 8** for risk factors
	Pregnant women	Screen	First trimester Third trimester if increased risk	Test with HBsAg
	Men	Screen if at increased risk	No recommended intervals	See **Table 8** for risk factors
	MSM	Screen	One time	Test with HBsAg
	Persons with HIV	Screen	One time	Screen with HBsAg, anti-HBc, and/or anti-HBs
Hepatitis C	All persons born between 1945 and 1965	Screen	Once	
	Women	Screen if at increased risk	No recommended intervals	See **Table 9** for risk factors
	Pregnant women	No current recommendation but this is under review		
	Men	Screen if at increased risk	No recommended intervals	See **Table 9** for risk factors
	Persons with HIV	Screen	At initial presentation	
	MSM with HIV	Screen	Annually	

Data from Refs.[49–51]

Table 8
Risk behaviors and risk exposures for hepatitis B and C

Hepatitis C	Hepatitis B

1. Current or past injection drug use
2. Long-term hemodialysis
3. Born to hepatitis C–infected mother
4. Incarceration
5. Intranasal drug use
6. Unregulated tattoo
7. Multiple sex partners
8. Sex with hepatitis C–infected person or injection drug user
9. Received blood products or underwent organ transplantation before July 1992
10. Received clotting factor concentrates produced before 1987
11. HIV infection
12. About to start PrEP for HIV
	• Active injection drug users
	• MSM
	• Patients receiving hemodialysis, cytotoxic or immunosuppressive therapy
	• Not vaccinated
	• Foreign born persons or their unvaccinated children whose country of origin has a high prevalence (>8%) of hepatitis B such as sub-Saharan Africa, central and southeast Asia, and China
	• Patients in high-risk settings, such as:
	  ○ Correctional facilities
	  ○ Institutions that serve populations from countries with a high prevalence of infection
	  ○ Community health centers
	  ○ STD clinics

Data from Refs.[49–51]

Table 9
Interpretation of the hepatitis B serologic panel

Interpretation	HbsAg	Anti-HBc	Anti-HBs
Immune due to history of infection	Negative	Positive	Positive
Immune due to hepatitis B vaccination	Negative	Negative	Positive
Susceptible to hepatitis B infection[a]	Negative	Negative	Negative
Infected[b]	Positive	Positive	Negative

[a] Patients with this result should be referred for hepatitis B vaccination. If they have had hepatitis B vaccination series twice, they may be a nonresponder.
[b] Patients who are infected may need further serologic testing to determine acute vs chronic infections.
Data from Mast EE, Margolis HS, Fiore AE, et al. A comprehensive immunization strategy to eliminate transmission of hepatitis B virus infection in the United States: recommendations of the Advisory Committee on Immunization Practices. Part I: immunization of infants, children, and adolescents. MMWR Recomm Rep 2005;54(No. RR-16):1–31.

Treatment

Treatment of these diseases is rapidly changing and outside the scope of this article. Please see current guidelines from the CDC.

Trichomonas

USPSTF does not have a recommendation for screening asymptomatic patients for trichomonas. The CDC recommends screening in HIV-positive women at presentation and then annually. They also recommend screening in high-risk/high-prevalence settings, such as correctional facilities and STD clinics.[52]

Herpes Simplex Virus 1 and 2

Herpes is one of the most prevalent STIs. Almost half of the population is infected with herpes simplex virus 1 (HSV1), and about 12% have herpes simplex virus 2 (HSV2).[53] HSV1 can be an oral or genital infection, and HSV2 is mostly a genital infection.[53] There is no cure for HSV. Treatment of HSV is primarily symptomatic, and there have been no good studies showing that screening asymptomatic individuals for HSV prevents sequelae or transmission. The USPSTF currently recommends against screening all asymptomatic individuals, including pregnant women.[54] The risks of false positive results, patient anxiety and relationship problems, and unnecessary antiviral medication outweigh the small benefit.[54]

SUMMARY

Sex is an important part of life. The goal for screening is to identify people at risk and mitigate those risks as much as possible. Screen all patients for risk factors for STIs. If the patient does have a risk factor, screen them for the infections they are at risk for. The trend in testing has been toward less invasive methods, such as vaginal self-swabs for gonorrhea and chlamydia.[55] The use of less invasive methods increases the number of people willing to undergo testing without decreasing the sensitivity of testing.[55] Always be mindful of the stigma that can come from being diagnosed with an STI and treat all patients with respect and dignity. Because the incidence and prevalence of specific STIs change in the general population, screening recommendations change as well. Always check the most updated recommendations when making screening and treatment decisions.

ACKNOWLEDGMENTS

The authors acknowledge Taria Poteat, MPH for her help in preparing this article.

REFERENCES

1. CDC Fact Sheet. Incidence, prevalence, and cost of sexually transmitted infections in the United States. February 2013. Available at: https://www.cdc.gov/std/stats/sti-estimates-fact-sheet-feb-2013.pdf.
2. Centers for Disease Control and Prevention. Sexually transmitted disease surveillance 2016. Atlanta (GA): U.S. Department of Health and Human Services; 2017.
3. Chlamydia screening data, HEDIS and managed care. Centers for Disease Control and Prevention; 2017. Available at: https://www.cdc.gov/std/chlamydia/hedis.htm. Accessed April 26, 2018.
4. A guide to taking a sexual history. Available at: www.cdc.gov. https://www.cdc.gov/std/treatment/sexualhistory.pdf. Accessed April 2, 2018.
5. 2016 sexually transmitted diseases surveillance. Centers for Disease Control and Prevention; 2017. Available at: https://www.cdc.gov/std/stats16/Gonorrhea.htm. Accessed April 2, 2018.
6. Zakher B, Cantor AG, Pappas M, et al. Screening for chlamydia and gonorrhea: U.S. Preventive Services Task Force recommendation statement. Ann Intern Med 2014;161(12). https://doi.org/10.7326/p14-9042.
7. MMWR. Elizabeth Torrone et al. September 26, 2014. Prevalence of chlamydia trachomatis genital infection among persons aged 14–39 Years — United States, 2007–2012. Available at: https://www.cdc.gov/mmwr/preview/mmwrhtml/mm6338a3.htm. Accessed April 2, 2018.
8. Chlamydia and gonorrhea: screening. final update summary: chlamydia and gonorrhea: screening - US Preventive Services Task Force. Available at: https://www.uspreventiveservicestaskforce.org/Page/Document/UpdateSummaryFinal/chlamydia-and-gonorrhea-screening. Accessed March 28, 2018.
9. Screening recommendations and considerations referenced in treatment guidelines and original sources. Centers for Disease Control and Prevention; 2016. Available at: https://www.cdc.gov/std/tg2015/screening-recommendations.htm. Accessed February 15, 2018.
10. Women's Health Care Physicians. Sexually transmitted infections: resource overview - ACOG. Available at: https://www.acog.org/Womens-Health/Sexually-Transmitted-Infections. Accessed April 11, 2018.
11. Committee on Adolescence and Society for Adolescent Health and Medicine. Screening for nonviral sexually transmitted infections in adolescents and young adults. Pediatrics 2014;134(1):e302–11. Available at: http://pediatrics.aappublications.org/content/134/1/e302. Accessed March 7, 2018.
12. Lee KC, Ngo-Metzger Q, Wolff T, et al. Sexually transmitted infections: recommendations from the U.S. Preventive Services Task Force. Am Fam Physician 2016;94(11):907–15. Available at: https://www.aafp.org/afp/2016/1201/p907.html. Accessed March 20, 2018.
13. US Preventive Services Task Force (USPSTF). Screening for syphilis infection in nonpregnant adults and adolescents US Preventive Services Task Force recommendation statement. JAMA 2016;315(21):2321–7.
14. Yang B, Hallmark CJ, Huang JS, et al. Characteristics and risk of syphilis diagnosis among HIV-infected male cohort: a population-based study in Houston, Texas. Sex Transm Dis 2013;40(12):957–63.

15. Oakeshott P, Kerry S, Aghaizu A, et al. Randomised controlled trial of screening for Chlamydia trachomatis to prevent pelvic inflammatory disease: the POPI (prevention of pelvic infection) trial. BMJ 2010;340:c1642.

16. 2015 sexually transmitted diseases treatment guidelines. Centers for Disease Control and Prevention; 2018. Available at: https://www.cdc.gov/std/tg2015/gonorrhea.htm. Accessed March 28, 2018.

17. Centers for Disease Control and Prevention. Sexually transmitted diseases (STDs). Syphilis – CDC Fact Sheet. 2017. Available at: https://www.cdc.gov/std/syphilis/stdfact-syphilis.htm. Accessed December 27, 2017.

18. Centers for Disease Control and Prevention. Sexually transmitted disease surveillance, 2014. 2015. Available at: http://www.cdc.gov. Accessed April 22, 2018.

19. Centers for Disease Control and Prevention. Division of STD Prevention. Recommendations for public health surveillance of syphilis in the United States. 2018. Available at: http://www.cdc.gov/std/syphsurvreco.pdf. Accessed April 18, 2018.

20. The American College of Obstetricians and Gynecologists, Womens Healthcare Physicians. Chlamydia, Gonorrhea, and Syphilis. FAQ071, December 2016. Available at: https://www.acog.org/Patients/FAQs/Chlamydia-Gonorrhea-and-Syphilis#syphilis. Accessed April 17, 2018.

21. Mattei PI, Beachkofsky TM, Gilson RT, et al. Syphilis: a reemerging infection. Am Fam Physician 2012;86(5):433–40.

22. Centers for Disease and Prevention. 2015 sexually transmitted diseases treatment guidelines. congenital syphilis. 2015. Available at: https://www.cdc.gov/std/tg2015/congenital.htm. Accessed April 18, 2018.

23. Bolan G, STD Prevention, National Center, TB Prevention, Centers for Disease Control and Prevention. Syphilis and HIV: a dangerous duo affecting gay and bisexual men. HIV.gov. 2018. Available at: https://www.hiv.gov/blog/syphilis-and-hiv-a-dangerous-duo-affecting-gay-and-bisexual-men. Accessed May 1, 2018.

24. Syphilis during pregnancy. Centers for Disease Control and Prevention; 2016. Available at: https://www.cdc.gov/std/tg2015/syphilis-pregnancy.htm. Accessed April 23, 2018.

25. Goh BT. Syphilis in adults. Sexually Transmitted Infections. 2005. Available at: http://sti.bmj.com/content/81/6/448.full. Accessed April 27, 2018.

26. Van Dyck E, Meheus AZ, Piot P. Syphilis. In: Laboratory diagnosis of sexually transmitted diseases. Geneva (Switzerland): World Health Organization; 1999. p. 36–49. Available at: http://apps.who.int/iris/handle/10665/41847. Accessed April 27, 2018.

27. Robinson A. Screening for syphilis with a treponemal enzyme immunoassay. Test updates. Paclab Network Laboratories; 2010. Available at: https://www.paclab.com/Files/TestUpdates/Syphilis%20PACLAB.pdf.

28. Creegan L, Bauer HM, Samuel MC, et al. An evaluation of the relative sensitivities of the venereal disease research laboratory test and the Treponema Pallidum particle agglutination test among patients diagnosed with primary syphilis. Sex Transm Dis 2007;34:1016–108.

29. Manavi K, Young H, McMillan A. The sensitivity of syphilis assays in detecting different stages of early syphilis. Int J STD AIDS 2006;17:768–71.

30. CDC STD Guidelines and Recommendations | National Prevention Information Network. Centers for Disease Control and Prevention. Available at: https://npin.cdc.gov/pages/cdc-std-guidelines-and-recommendations. Accessed April 27, 2018.

31. Syphilis. Centers for Disease Control and Prevention; 2016. Available at: https://www.cdc.gov/std/tg2015/syphilis.htm. Accessed April 23, 2018.

32. Brown DL, Frank JE. Diagnosis and management of syphilis. Am Fam Physician 2003;62(2):283–90. Accessed April 27, 2018. https://www.aafp.org/afp/2003/0715/p283.html.

33. Centers for Disease Control and Prevention. HIV in the United States: at a glance. 2017. Available at: https://www.cdc.gov/hiv/statistics/overview/ataglance.html. Accessed April 22, 2018.

34. World Health Organization. HIV/AIDS, fact sheet. 2017. Available at: http://www.who.int/mediacentre/factsheets/fs360/en/. Accessed on April 12, 2018.

35. Chu C, Selwyn PA, Einstein A. Diagnosis and initial management of acute HIV infection. Am Fam Physician 2010;81(10):1239–44.

36. Committee on Pediatric AIDS, Emmanuel PJ, Martinez J. Adolescents and HIV infection: the pediatrician's role in promoting routine testing. Pediatrics 2011; 128(5):1023–9.

37. Centers for Disease Control and Prevention. HIV among men in the United States. MSM testing initiatives. 2017. Available at: https://www.cdc.gov/hiv/group/gender/men/index.html. Accessed April 22, 2018.

38. The American College of Obstetricians and Gynecologists, Women's Healthcare Physicians. Clinical guidelines: perinatal screening. Number 635, June 2015. Available at: https://www.acog.org/Clinical-Guidance-and-Publications/Committee-Opinions/Committee-on-Obstetric-Practice/Prenatal-and-Perinatal-Human-Immunodeficiency-Virus-Testing-Expanded-Recommendations. Accessed April 18, 2018.

39. United States Preventive Services Task Force. Screening for Human Immunodeficiency Virus (HIV) April 2013. 2016. Available at: https://www.uspreventiveservicestaskforce.org/Home/GetFileByID/1890. Accessed April 12, 2018.

40. National HIV Curriculum. HIV screening recommendations. Rational for routine HIV screening. 2017. Available at: https://www.hiv.uw.edu/go/screening-diagnosis/recommendations-testing/core-concept/all. Accessed April 22, 2018.

41. Centers for Disease Control and Prevention. Stages of HIV infection. HIV risk reduction tool. 2018. Available at: https://wwwn.cdc.gov/hivrisk/what_is/stages_hiv_infection.html. Accessed April 20, 2018.

42. HIV/AIDS. Centers for Disease Control and Prevention; 2018. Available at: https://www.cdc.gov/hiv/risk/prep/index.html. Accessed June 20, 2018.

43. Welcome to CDC stacks | 2018 Quick reference guide: recommended laboratory HIV testing algorithm for serum or plasma specimens - 50872 | Guidelines and Recommendations. Centers for Disease Control and Prevention. Available at: https://stacks.cdc.gov/view/cdc/50872. Accessed April 29, 2018.

44. Welcome to CDC stacks | Laboratory testing for the diagnosis of HIV infection : updated recommendations - 23447 | Guidelines and recommendations. Centers for Disease Control and Prevention. Available at: https://stacks.cdc.gov/view/cdc/23447. Accessed April 29, 2018.

45. What is hepatitis? World Health Organization; 2017. Available at: http://www.who.int/features/qa/76/en/. Accessed April 29, 2018.

46. Viral hepatitis. Centers for Disease Control and Prevention; 2018. Available at: https://www.cdc.gov/hepatitis/statistics/2016surveillance/commentary.htm. Accessed May 1, 2018.

47. Viral hepatitis. Centers for Disease Control and Prevention; 2015. Available at: https://www.cdc.gov/hepatitis/hbv/index.htm. Accessed May 1, 2018.

48. Tsoulfas G, Goulis I, Giakoustidis D, et al. Hepatitis C and liver transplantation. Hippokratia 2009;13(4):211–5.

49. Hepatitis B Virus Infection: Screening, 2014. Final update summary: hepatitis B virus infection: screening, 2014 - US Preventive Services Task Force. Available at: https://www.uspreventiveservicestaskforce.org/Page/Document/Update SummaryFinal/hepatitis-b-virus-infection-screening-2014. Accessed April 6, 2018.

50. Hepatitis C: screening. Final update summary: hepatitis C: screening - US Preventive Services Task Force. Available at: https://www.uspreventiveservicestaskforce. org/Page/Document/UpdateSummaryFinal/hepatitis-c-screening. Accessed April 13, 2018.

51. HCV in Pregnancy | HCV guidance. Available at: https://www.hcvguidelines.org/ unique-populations/pregnancy. Accessed April 10, 2018.

52. Screening recommendations and considerations referenced in treatment guidelines and original sources. Centers for Disease Control and Prevention; 2016. Available at: https://www.cdc.gov/std/tg2015/screening-recommendations.htm. Accessed April 27, 2018.

53. National Center for Health Statistics. Centers for Disease Control and Prevention. 2018. Available at: https://www.cdc.gov/nchs/products/databriefs/db304.htm. Accessed April 27, 2018.

54. US Preventive Services Task Force. Serologic screening for genital herpes infection. US Preventive Services Task Force recommendation statement. JAMA 2016; 316(23):2525–30.

55. Stewart CMW, Schoeman SA, Booth RA, et al. Assessment of self taken swabs versus clinician taken swab cultures for diagnosing gonorrhoea in women: single centre, diagnostic accuracy study. BMJ 2012;345. https://doi.org/10.1136/bmj. e8107.

Update on Osteoporosis

Srikala Yedavally-Yellayi, DO, MEd[a,b],*, Andrew Manyin Ho, DO[a],
Erwin Matthew Patalinghug, MD[a]

KEYWORDS

- Screening • DEXA • Low bone mass • Bisphosphonates • Osteoporosis
- Bone mineral density

KEY POINTS

- Osteoporosis and low bone mass pose significant disease burden on America's growing older population.
- Decreasing bone mass and microarchitectural deterioration lead to increased fracture risk characterize osteoporosis.
- Screening guidelines using bone mineral density testing vary by expert group, but assessing fracture risk in vulnerable populations is a universal recommendation.
- Risk factor assessment with modification along with pharmacologic treatment is recommended to reduce fracture risk and subsequently morbidity and mortality.
- Monitoring during pharmacologic treatment is recommended; however, there is no consensus on monitoring frequency.

CLINICAL DESCRIPTION OF DISEASE

America is an aging nation. By 2060, America's population of adults over the age of 65 is expected to double the current number to 98 million people.[1] Aging increases the prevalence of low bone mass and microarchitectural deterioration of bone, resulting in osteoporosis.

Definition

Osteoporosis is a skeletal disorder characterized by reduced bone mineral density (BMD) and mass, resulting in damaged bone structure. Decreased density can occur when the body loses too much bone, makes too little bone, or both. As a result, there is a reduction in bone strength, which manifests clinically when bones fracture.[2] Factors that contribute to skeletal fragility include aging, genetics, nutrition, vitamin and

Disclosure Statement: The authors have nothing to disclose.
[a] Department of Family Medicine, Family Medicine Residency Program, Beaumont Health Troy, 44250 Dequindre Road, Sterling Heights, MI 48314, USA; [b] Oakland University William Beaumont School of Medicine, O'Dowd Hall, 586 Pioneer Drive, Rochester, MI 48309, USA
* Corresponding author.
E-mail address: Srikala.yedavally@beaumont.edu

Prim Care Clin Office Pract 46 (2019) 175–190
https://doi.org/10.1016/j.pop.2018.10.014
0095-4543/19/© 2018 Elsevier Inc. All rights reserved.

primarycare.theclinics.com

mineral deficiency, lifestyle choices, smoking history, hormonal production, and medications. To help define osteoporosis, the World Health Organization has categorized changes in BMD) into 4 groups based on dual-energy x-ray absorptiometry (DEXA) T score: normal (+1 to −1), low bone mass or osteopenia (−1 to −2.5), osteoporosis (−2.5 to −3),[3] and severe osteoporosis (BMD T score of −2.5 or below plus a fragility fracture, or T score of −3.5 or below in the absence of fractures).[4]

Pathology

Bone is an active tissue that constantly remodels itself in response to mechanical stress and hormonal changes. The process of bone remodeling begins with bone resorption, during which osteoclasts digest old bone. The next phase is reversal, where mononuclear cells appear on the bone surface. The final phase is formation, when osteoblasts lay down new bone until resorbed bone is completely replaced.[5] This bone remodeling is regulated by numerous cytokines, including interleukins 1, 6, and 11. Additional factors, such as parathyroid hormone, Vitamin D, calcitonin, and estrogen, are known to stimulate bone growth.[6] Factors that stimulate osteoclast bone resorption include tumor necrosis factor, receptor activator of nuclear factor kappa B, and insulin growth factor-1 (**Fig. 1**). An imbalance in these factors results in poor bone remodeling, which is then seen on imaging as lower bone density.

Clinically, osteoporosis is a silent disease, because weak bones are not painful until a fracture occurs. Many patients without symptoms incorrectly assume that they do

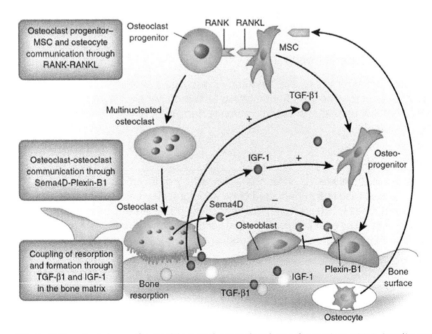

Fig. 1. Pathophysiology of osteoblast and osteoclast bone formation. IGF-1, insulin growth factor-1; MSC, mesenchymal stem cell; RANK, receptor activator of nuclear factor kappa B; RANKL, receptor activator of nuclear factor kappa B ligand; TNF, tumor necrosis factor. (*From* Cao X. Targeting osteoclast-osteoblast communication. Nat Med 2011;17:1344–6; with permission.)

not have osteoporosis. Contrarily, patients with joint pain and a lack of fracture will incorrectly assume that they have osteoporosis. As such, it is important for a family physician to help patients differentiate between symptoms and a diagnosis of osteoporosis.

EPIDEMIOLOGY

The National Osteoporosis Foundation, based on data from the National Health and Nutrition Examination Survey III, estimates more than 9.9 million Americans have osteoporosis and an additional 43.1 million have low bone density **(Fig. 2)**.[7] Annually, more than 1.5 million osteoporosis-related fractures occur in the United States, the vast majority occurring in women.[8] In addition, it is estimated up to 25% of men over the age of 50 will experience a fracture due to osteoporosis.[9] In fact, approximately 50% of Americans older than 50 years of age are at risk for osteoporotic fracture With an estimated economic burden on the health care system of US$25.3 billion per year by 2025.[10]

Given the high disease burden based on the projections of an aging population in the United States, screening for osteoporosis can have significant long-term impact because osteoporosis is a disease that can be prevented, diagnosed, and treated before fractures occur.[7] Screening includes assessment of risk factors for fractures

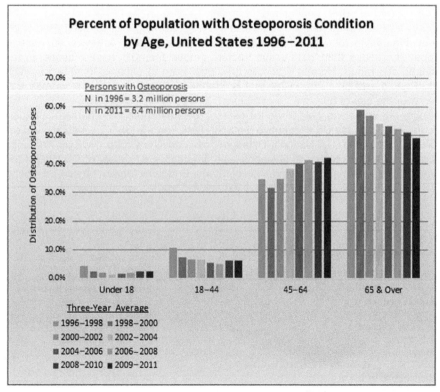

Fig. 2. Prevalence of osteoporosis in the United States. (*Reprinted with permission of* the World Health Organization Collaborating Centre for Metabolic Bone Diseases, University of Sheffield Medical School, UK.)

as well as using BMD measurement using DEXA. Validated risk factors for fracture prediction, independent of BMD, include advanced age, previous fracture, long-term glucocorticoid therapy, low body weight (less than 58 kg), family history of hip fracture, cigarette smoking, and excess alcohol intake.[11] It is recommended to assess risk factors for fracture in all adults, especially postmenopausal women, men over the age of 50 years, and any person who experiences a fragility fracture of low-trauma fracture.[12]

Understanding modifiable and nonmodifiable risk factors for osteoporosis is also important in overall risk factor assessment. Although certain risk factors are fixed or nonmodifiable, those risk factors that are modifiable provide opportunities for physicians to educate and counsel patients on lifestyle changes that can mitigate the impact of certain behaviors. Assessing risk factors for falls is also important because most osteoporosis-related fractures result from falls (**Table 1**).[7]

Consideration of these risk factors may trigger BMD testing at an earlier age than currently recommended. However, it is important to note that fracture risk is greater in the presence of specific risk factors than can be accounted for with BMD testing alone (see **Fig. 2**).[13] Therefore, fracture risk assessment should take into account the impact of these risk factors in addition to BMD testing.[13] In 2008, the Fracture Risk Assessment Tool (FRAX), an online algorithm, was developed, using specific risk factors, with and without T scores, to estimate the 10-year probability of hip fracture and the 10-year probability of a major osteoporotic fracture (spine, forearm, hip, or shoulder fracture).[14] It has been validated in more than 40 cohorts and can provide guidance for both BMD testing and treatment.[12] Although the FRAX tool is not a substitute for clinical judgment, it can aid in identifying patients for BMD testing and treatment (**Fig. 3**). In fact, most patients with a 10-year major osteoporotic fracture probability greater than 20% or hip fracture greater than 3% have T scores in the osteoporotic range. Normal T scores are rarely seen in patients identified as high risk (**Figs. 4** and **5**).[15] The FRAX tool is intended for postmenopausal women and men over the age of 50.[7]

There are screening guidelines for osteoporosis available from numerous expert groups, including the US Preventive Services Task Force (USPSTF), National Osteoporosis Foundation, UK National Osteoporosis Guideline Group (NOGG), American College of Obstetricians and Gynecologists, International Society of Clinical Densitometry, and the American Association of Clinical Endocrinologists. Most recommend BMD testing of the hip and/or spine except for NOGG, which does not endorse

Table 1	
Nonmodifiable and modifiable risk factors	
Fixed (Nonmodifiable) Risk Factors	**Modifiable Risk Factors**
Age	Excessive alcohol consumption
Female gender	Smoking
Family history	Low BMI
Previous fracture	Poor nutrition
Ethnicity	Vitamin D deficiency
Menopause or hysterectomy	Eating disorders
Long-term glucocorticoid therapy	Estrogen deficiency
Rheumatoid arthritis	Insufficient exercise
Primary or secondary hypogonadism in men	

From International Osteoporosis Foundation. Available at: https://www.iofbonehealth.org. Accessed January 30, 2018.

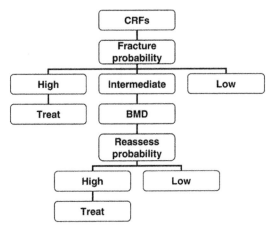

Fig. 3. Management algorithm for the assessment of individuals at risk of fracture. CRF, corticotropin-releasing factor. (*Reprinted with permission of* the World Health Organization Collaborating Centre for Metabolic Bone Diseases, University of Sheffield Medical School, UK.)

population screening but recommends fracture risk assessment in postmenopausal women using the FRAX tool. In the United States, most expert groups recommend BMD testing, using DEXA for women aged 65 years and older regardless of clinical risk factors (**Table 2**). Recommendations on screening for women under the age of 65 and older men vary and are based on a variety of risk factors for bone loss and osteoporosis. For example, to screen women between the ages of 50 and 64 years,

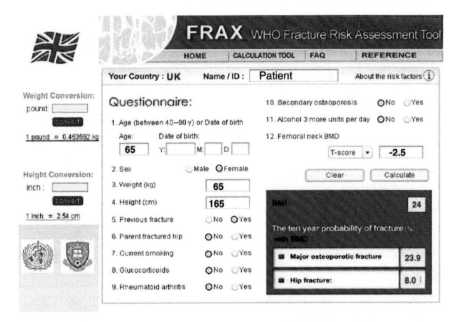

Fig. 4. Chart for input of data and format of results in the UK version of the FRAX tool. (*Courtesy of* the World Health Organization Collaborating Centre for Metabolic Bone Diseases, University of Sheffield Medical School, UK; with permission.)

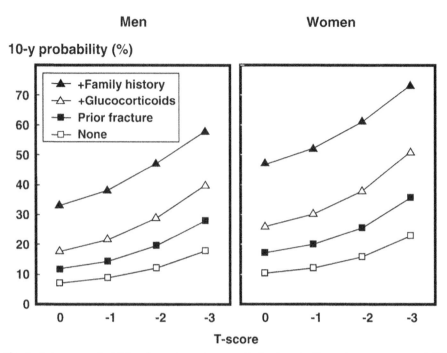

Fig. 5. Ten-year probability of a major osteoporotic fracture in Caucasian women aged 65 years from the United States according to the presence of the clinical risk factors shown. The BMI is set at 24 kg/m^2. (*From* Kanis JA, Oden A, Johansson H, et al. FRAX and its applications to clinical practice. Bone 2009;44(5):736; with permission.)

USPSTF recommends using a 10-year fracture risk threshold of 9.3% bearing in mind clinical judgment (see **Table 2**). In addition, annual height measurement is recommended, preferably using a wall-mounted stadiometer.[7] Biochemical markers of bone remodeling are available and used clinically; however, their utility in the algorithm for BMD testing and screening for osteoporosis remains unknown.[7]

Once screening is initiated, there is a paucity of evidence for optimal intervals for rescreening.[7] However, the National Osteoporosis Foundation, in accordance with Medicare guidelines, recommends repeat BMD assessment every 2 years, understanding the interval may change based on the clinical situation.[7] In addition, vertebral imaging should be performed in postmenopausal women and men aged 50 and older with the following risk factors[7]:

1. A low-trauma fracture during adulthood defined as aged 50 and older
2. Historical height loss described as the difference between current height and peak height at age of 20 of 4 cm or more
3. Prospective height loss described as the difference between the current height and a previously documented height measurement of 2 cm or more
4. Recent or ongoing long-term glucocorticoid treatment
5. If bone density testing is unavailable, may be considered based on age alone

Vertebral imaging is also indicated in patients who meet the following criteria:

1. In all women aged 70 and older and all men aged 80 and older if BMD T score is less than or equal to −1.0 at the spine, total hip, or femoral neck.

Table 2
Screening recommendations

Organization	Recommendations	
	Women	**Men**
National Osteoporosis Foundation (NOF)[7]	DEXA testing for all women >65 y old and postmenopausal women <65 y old, based on risk factor profile, younger postmenopausal women, women in menopausal transition	DEXA testing for all men >70 y old, regardless of risk factor profile, and men age 50–69 y old with clinical risk factors for fracture
	• DEXA testing for adults who have a fracture after age 50 y	
	• DEXA testing for adults with a condition (eg, rheumatoid arthritis) or taking a medication (eg, glucocorticoids in a daily dose ≥5 mg prednisone or equivalent for ≥3 mo) associated with low bone mass or bone loss	
US Preventive Services Task Force (USPSTF)[29]	• BMD testing for all women>65 y old	Insufficient evidence to assess the balance of benefits and harms of screening in men
	• BMD testing in women younger than 65 y old who are at increased risk osteoporosis as determined by a formal clinical risk assessment tool	
UK National Osteoporosis Guidelines Group (NOGG)[30]	Does not recommend population screening	Fracture probability should be assessed in men >50 y who have risk factors for fracture using FRAX
	Fracture probability should be assessed in postmenopausal women using FRAX	
	• In individuals at intermediate risk, BMD testing using DEXA should be performed and fracture probability reassessed using FRAX.	
	• Vertebral fracture assessment should be considered in postmenopausal women and men age >50 y if there is a history of ≥4 cm height loss, kyphosis, recent or current long-term oral glucocorticoid therapy, or a BMD T score of ≤2.5	
American Academy of Pain Medicine (AAPM) American Association of Clinical Endocrinologists (AACE) American Orthopaedic Association (AOA) American Society for Bone and Mineral Research (ASBMR) International Society for Clinical Densitometry (ISCD)	• Measure height annually • NOF guidelines (as above) • Vertebral imaging in special populations (as above)	

Adapted from US Preventive Services Task Force. Screening for osteoporosis: US Preventive Services Task Force recommendation statement. Ann Intern Med 2011;154(5):362; with permission.

2. In women aged 65 to 69 and men aged 70 to 79 if BMD T score is less than −1% at the spine, total hip, or femoral neck.

Quantitative sonography of the calcaneus is an acceptable and more affordable alternative because it predicts fractures of the hip, spine, and femoral neck equivalent to DEXA, but it is important to note current diagnostic and treatment criteria for osteoporosis are based on DEXA measurements only.[16]

Special Populations

Screening in men
The most important risk factors for low BMD-associated osteoporotic fractures are age greater than 70 years and low body weight, body mass index (BMI) less than 20 to 25 kg/m^2.[17]

Screening in younger populations
There is no evidence for screening populations under the age of 50 unless there are significant risk factors as outlined in **Table 1**. Adolescents should be evaluated for risk behaviors that may lead to osteoporosis. During adolescence, lifestyle habits are forming, and it is a stage of bone building. Lifestyle interventions to curb tobacco and alcohol use as well as establishing a daily exercise regimen can have meaningful long-term impact.[18]

Potential Harms of Screening

Although benefits of screening are apparent in that early diagnosis may help prevent future morbidity and decrease mortalities from fracture complications, it is important to note potential harms from screening:

1. False positive test results, which lead to unnecessary treatment
2. False negative test results, where treatment is not rendered when needed
3. Patient anxiety associated with positive test results

Secondary Causes of Osteoporosis

Several disease states as well as chronic medication use can contribute to the development of osteoporosis[19] (**Table 3**). Laboratory testing can be helpful and is indicated in ruling out these disease states as the cause of osteoporosis (**Box 1**).[19]

PREVENTION RECOMMENDATIONS

Prevention is considered a mainstay for management of osteoporosis and the associated sequelae. Patients are sometimes identified early with osteopenia. Multiple societies endorse a comprehensive patient evaluation.

All postmenopausal women and men older than 50 should receive counseling. This discussion should include the risks of osteoporosis and associated fractures.[7] Early assessment of secondary causes and risk factors is recommended. Lifestyle should be assessed, and modifications should be made as appropriate.[11] **Table 1** summarizes recommended risk factors to review.

Vitamin D and calcium supplementation can be recommended because deficiencies in these are known risk factors for osteoporosis. If these values cannot be obtained through diet, then supplementation should be considered. **Table 4** reviews daily recommended intake values.[7] Despite these recommendations though, data for an overall effect are lacking for both vitamin D and calcium.[10]

Physical activity is also recommended for prevention of progression of bone disease. Weight-bearing and muscle-strengthening exercise programs should be discussed with goals of improving safe movement, maintaining bone

Table 3
Conditions, diseases, and medications that cause or contribute to osteoporosis and fractures

Lifestyle factors

Alcohol abuse	Excessive thinness	Excess vitamin A
Frequent falling	High salt intake	Immobilization
Inadequate physical activity	Low calcium intake	Smoking (active or passive)
Vitamin D insufficiency		

Genetic diseases

Cystic fibrosis	Ehlers-Danlos	Gaucher disease
Glycogen storage diseases	Hemochromatosis	Homocystinuria
Hypophosphatasia	Marfan syndrome	Menkes steely hair syndrome
Osteogenesis imperfecta	Parental history of hip	Porphyria
Riley-Day syndrome	fracture	

Hypogonadal states

Androgen insensitivity	Anorexia nervosa	Athletic amenorrhea
Hyperprolactinemia	Panhypopituitarism	Premature menopause
Turner and Klinefelter		(<40 y)
syndromes		

Endocrine disorders

Central obesity	Cushing syndrome	Diabetes mellitus
Hyperparathyroidism	Thyrotoxicosis	(types 1 and 2)

Gastrointestinal disorders

Celiac disease	Gastric bypass	Gastrointestinal surgery
Inflammatory bowel disease	Malabsorption	Pancreatic disease
Primary biliary cirrhosis		

Hematologic disorders

Hemophilia	Leukemia and lymphomas	Monoclonal gammopathies
Multiple myeloma	Sickle cell disease	Systemic mastocytosis
Thalassemia		

Rheumatologic and autoimmune diseases

Ankylosing spondylitis	Other rheumatic and	
Rheumatoid arthritis	autoimmune diseases	
	Systemic lupus	

Neurologic and musculoskeletal risk factors

Epilepsy	Multiple sclerosis	Muscular dystrophy
Parkinson disease	Spinal cord injury	Stroke

Miscellaneous conditions and diseases

AIDS/HIV	Amyloidosis	Chronic metabolic acidosis
Chronic obstructive lung disease	Congestive heart failure	Depression
End-stage renal disease	Hypercalciuria	Idiopathic scoliosis
Posttransplant bone disease	Sarcoidosis	Weight loss

Medications

Aluminum (in antacids)	Anticoagulants (heparin)	Anticonvulsants
Aromatase inhibitors	Barbiturates	Cancer chemotherapeutic
Depo-medroxyprogesterone	Glucocorticoids	drugs
(premenopausal	(≥5 mg/d prednisone	GnRH (gonadotropin-
contraception)	or equivalent for ≥3 mo)	releasing hormone)
Lithium cyclosporine A and	Methotrexate	agonists
tacrolimus	Selective serotonin	Parental nutrition
Proton pump inhibitors	reuptake inhibitors	Thyroid hormones (in excess)
Tamoxifen (premenopausal use)	Thiazolidinediones (such as	
	Actos and Avandia)	

From Cosman F, de Beur SJ, LeBoff MS, et al. Clinician's guide to prevention and treatment of osteoporosis. Osteoporos Int 2014;25(10):2364; with permission.

Box 1
Exclusion of secondary causes of osteoporosis

Consider the following diagnostic studies for secondary causes of osteoporosis

Blood or serum
  Complete blood count
  Chemistry levels (calcium, renal function, phosphorus, and magnesium)
  Liver function tests
  Thyroid-stimulating hormone ± free T_4
  25(OH)D
  Parathyroid hormone
  Total testosterone and gonadotropin in younger men
  Bone turnover markers

Consider in selected patients
  Serum protein electrophoresis, serum immunofixation, serum-free light chains
  Tissue transglutaminase antibodies (IgA and IgG)
  Iron and ferritin levels
  Homocysteine
  Prolactin
  Tryptase

Urine
  24-h urinary calcium

Consider in selected patients
  Protein electrophoresis (UPEP)
  Urinary-free cortisol level
  Urinary histamine

From Cosman F, de Beur SJ, LeBoff MS, et al. Clinician's guide to prevention and treatment of osteoporosis. Osteoporos Int 2014;25(10):2366; with permission.

---

strength, and reducing fall/fracture risk.[7,20] Similarly, though, the current evidence is insufficient to show definitive impact of physical activity on fracture risk.[10]

The American Geriatric Society and Centers for Disease Control and Prevention (CDC) recommend patients older than 65 with osteoporosis be screened for fall risk. Subsequently, steps should be taken to prevent falls. Both the assessment and the plan can be implemented through a clinical algorithm (**Fig. 6**).[21]

When treatment is selected, there are many interventions that may impact the fracture risk of a patient. In addition to aforementioned risk management, pharmacotherapy can be considered. **Table 5** lists interventions that have been shown to

---

Table 4
Vitamin D and calcium intake recommendations

Vitamin D	
All individuals >50 y	800–1000 IU daily
Calcium	
Men 50–70 y old	1000 mg daily
Men 71 y and older	1200 mg daily
Women 51 y and older	1200 mg daily

Data from Cosman F, de Beur SJ, LeBoff MS, et al. Clinician's guide to prevention and treatment of osteoporosis. Osteoporos Int 2014;25(10):2359–81.

Algorithm for Fall Risk Screening, Assessment, and Intervention

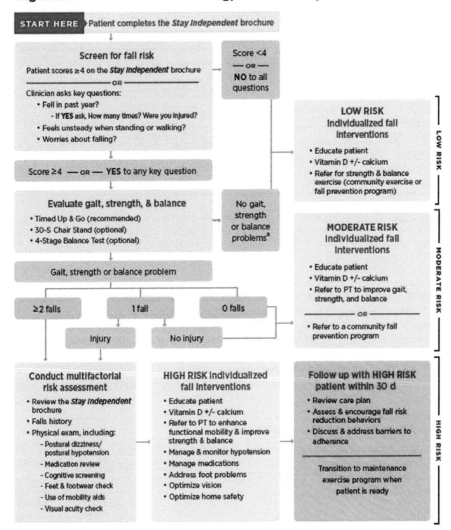

Fig. 6. STEADI CDC algorithm to assess fall risk and stratify patient. [a] For these patients, consider additional risk assessment (eg, medication review, cognitive screen, syncope). PT, physical therapy. (*From* Centers for Disease Control and Prevention. Resource algorithm for fall risk screening, assessment, and intervention. Available at: https://www.cdc.gov/steadi/pdf/STEADI-Algorithm-print.pdf. Accessed November 11, 2018.)

reduce fracture risk. First-line, Food and Drug Administration–approved pharmaco-therapy for osteoporosis typically includes oral bisphosphonates. Alendronate and risedronate are first-choice bisphosphonates because of their efficacy in reducing vertebral and hip fractures and favorable cost.[22] BMD monitoring is currently controversial with different societies not reaching consensus, as discussed in **Table 6**. For example, the National Osteoporosis Foundation recommends BMD monitoring 1 to 2 years after initiating medical therapy and every 2 years

Table 5
Pharmacologic treatments for osteoporosis/low bone density

	Fracture Risk		
Treatment	Vertebral	Nonvertebral	Hip
Alendronate	Improves	Improves	Improves
Ibandronate	Improves	Uncertain	Uncertain
Risedronate	Improves	Improves	Improves
Zoledronic acid	Improves	Improves	Improves
Denosumab	Improves	Improves	Improves
Teriparatide	Improves	Improves	Uncertain
Raloxifene	Improves	No effect	No effect
Calcium/vitamin D	Uncertain	Uncertain	Uncertain
Menopausal hormone therapy	Improves[a]	Uncertain	Improves

[a] Not beneficial in established osteoporosis.
From Qaseem A, Forciea MA, McLean RM, et al. Treatment of low bone density or osteoporosis to prevent fractures in men and women: a clinical practice guideline update from the American College of Physicians. Ann Intern Med 2017;166:825; with permission.

thereafter, which is in agreement with Medicare guidelines.[7] However, recent American College of Physicians literature recommends against monitoring during the first 5 years of treatment. Of note, this is a weak recommendation based on low-quality evidence.[10] Accurate yearly height measurement is a critical determination of osteoporosis treatment efficacy. Patients who lose 2 cm (or 0.8 inch) or more in height either acutely or cumulatively should have a repeat vertebral imaging test to determine if new or additional vertebral fractures have occurred since the prior vertebral imaging test.[23]

Outcomes for Patients and Complications

Bone loss itself is often asymptomatic. Fractures are the most common outcomes associated with osteoporosis.[24] In the United States, data for this primarily come from surveys belonging to CDC and Agency for Healthcare Research and Quality. Hip fractures and spinal fractures are most prevalent, but other common sites include

Table 6
Bone mineral density monitoring recommendations

American Academy of Family Physicians	"After initiation of treatment, the need for follow-up bone density testing is uncertain."[11]
American College of Physicians	"...recommends against bone density monitoring during the 5-y pharmacologic treatment period for osteoporosis in women."[10]
American College of Endocrinology	"Monitor serial changes in lumbar spine, total hip, femoral neck BMD."[31]
American Academy of Orthopaedic Surgeons	"...BMD density does not indicate other important components of bone strength."[20]
National Osteoporosis Foundation	"Perform BMD testing one to 2 years after initiating medical therapy for osteoporosis and every 2 years thereafter."[7]

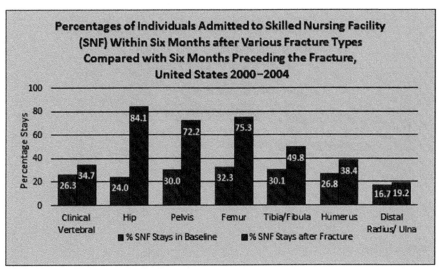

Fig. 7. Skilled nursing facility comparing the 6 months before and after various fracture types. (*From* United States Bone and Joint Initiative. The burden of musculoskeletal diseases in the United States (BMUS). 3rd edition. Rosemont (IL): United States Bone and Joint Initiative; 2014. Available at: http://www.boneandjointburden.org. Accessed April 10, 2018; with permission; and Becker DJ, Yun H, Kilgore ML, et al. Health services utilization after fractures: evidence from Medicare. J Gerontol A Biol Sci Med Sci 2010;65(9):1012–20.)

humerus, pelvis, femur, or wrist. These fractures often relate to a history of falling. Such fractures are often named "fragility fractures."

For example, between 2010 and 2011, approximately 4.3 million encounters for fragility fractures were noted in individuals over the age of 50 in the United States. This figure is inclusive of both inpatient and outpatient settings. Both osteoporosis and fragility fractures favor women nearly double to that of men. Age also plays a significant factor.[25]

Fractures have many consequences. Only approximately 40% of patients will regain prefracture level of function. Pain and activity limitations are commonly associated with fractures. There can also be psychosocial implications, such as depression. In addition, a history of fracture increases risk of another fracture.[11]

Fractures are associated with increased rate of hospitalization. After hospitalization, the disease process segues into higher probability of subsequent skilled nursing facilities use (**Fig. 7**) and ambulatory services use (physician visits, home visits, occupational therapy, and physical therapy).[26] Hip fractures, especially, are also associated with an increased risk of mortality and other comorbidities (**Fig. 8**).[27]

The mean cost per person with osteoporosis is US$10,978 from 2009 to 2011 (which increased 28% from 1996 to 1998). Consequently, the direct cost for persons with osteoporosis from 2009 to 2011 is approximately US$70.5 billion. The estimated cost associated with fractures is anticipated to be nearly US$25 billion by 2025, in part, due to population aging compared with US$18 billion in 2002.[28]

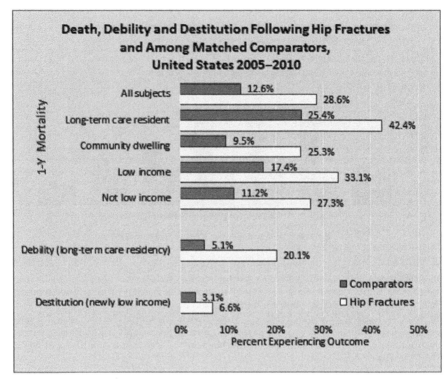

Fig. 8. Death, debility, and destitution in hip fracture patients compared with other Medicare beneficiaries. (*From* United States Bone and Joint Initiative. The burden of musculoskeletal diseases in the United States (BMUS). 3rd edition. Rosemont (IL): United States Bone and Joint Initiative; 2014. Available at:http://www.boneandjointburden.org. Accessed April 10, 2018; with permission; and Tajeu GS, Delzell E, Smith W, et al. Death, debility, and destitution following hip fracture. J Gerontol A Biol Sci Med Sci 2014;69(3):346–53.)

REFERENCES

1. Fact sheet: aging in the United States. Population Reference Bureau. Available at: https://www.prb.org/aging-unitedstates-fact-sheet/. Accessed April 28, 2018.

2. Learn what osteoporosis is and what it's caused by. National Osteoporosis Foundation. Available at: https://www.nof.org/patients/what-is-osteoporosis/. Accessed April 28, 2018.

3. World Health Organization. Topics & sites. Geneva (Switzerland): World Health Organization; 2016. Available at: http://www.who.int/chp/topics/en/ http://www.who.int/chp/topics/Osteoporosis.pdf. Accessed April 28, 2018.

4. Kendler DL, Marin F, Zerbini CA, et al. Effects of teriparatide and risedronate on new fractures in post-menopausal women with severe osteoporosis (VERO): a multicentre, double-blind, double-dummy, randomised controlled trial. Lancet 2018;391(10117):230–40. Available at: https://www.ncbi.nlm.nih.gov/pubmed?term=29129436. Accessed April 29, 2018.

5. Hadjidakis DJ, Androulakis II. Bone remodeling. Ann N Y Acad Sci 2006;1092:385–96. Available at: https://www.ncbi.nlm.nih.gov/pubmed/17308163. Accessed April 28, 2018.

6. Stavros C. Birth and death of bone cells: basic regulatory mechanisms and implications for the pathogenesis and treatment of osteoporosis * | Endocrine Reviews | Oxford Academic. OUP Academic, Oxford University Press; 2000. Available at: https://academic.oup.com/edrv/article/21/2/115/2423739.

7. Cosman F, de Beur SJ, LeBoff MS, et al. Clinician's guide to prevention and treatment of osteoporosis. Osteoporos Int 2014;25(10):2359–81.

8. U.S. Department of Health and Human Services. Bone Health and Osteoporosis: A Report of the Surgeon General. Rockville, MD: Office of the Surgeon General; 2004.

9. Sidlauskas KM, Sutton EE, Biddle MA. Osteoporosis in men: epidemiology and treatment with denosumab. Clin Interv Aging 2014;9:593–601.

10. Qaseem A, Forciea MA, McLean RM, et al. Treatment of low bone density or osteoporosis to prevent fractures in men and women: a clinical practice guideline update from the American College of Physicians. Ann Intern Med 2017;166(11): 818–39. Available at: http://annals.org/aim/fullarticle/2625385/treatment-low-bone-density-osteoporosis-prevent-fractures-men-women-clinical.

11. Jeremiah MP, Unwin BK, Greenawald MD, et al. Diagnosis and management of osteoporosis. Am Fam Physician 2015;92(4):261–8.

12. Yu EW. Screening for osteoporosis. In: Rosen CJ, SChmader kE, Mulder JE, editors. UptoDate. 2017. Available at: https://www.uptodate.com/contents/screening-for-osteoporosis.

13. Kanis JA, Oden A, Johansson H, et al. FRAX and its applications to clinical practice. Bone 2009;44(5):734–43.

14. University of Sheffield. Available at: https://www.sheffield.ac.uk/FRAX/tool.aspx?country=9. Accessed February 7, 2018.

15. Leslie WD, Majumdar SR, Lix LM, et al. High fracture probability with FRAX usually indicates densitometric osteoporosis: implications for clinical practice. Osteoporos Int 2012;23(1):391–7.

16. U.S. Preventive Services Task Force. Screening for osteoporosis: U.S. Preventive Services Task Force Recommendation Statement. Ann Intern Med 2011;154(5): 356–64.

17. Liu H, Paige NM, Goldzweig CL, et al. Screening for osteoporosis in men: a systematic review for an American College of Physicians Guideline. Ann Intern Med 2008;148(9):685–701.

18. Golden NH, Abrams SA, Committee on Nutrition. Optimizing bone health in children and adolescents. Pediatrics 2014;134(4):e1229–43.

19. Cosman F, de Beur SJ, LeBoff MS, et al. Clinician's guide to prevention and treatment of osteoporosis. Osteoporos Int 2014;25(10):2359–81.

20. American Academy of Orthopaedic Surgeons. Osteoporosis/Bone Health in Adults as a National Public Health Priority. 2014. Available at: http://www.aaos.org/About/Statements/Position/. Accessed April 10, 2018.

21. American Geriatric Society. Clinical practice guideline falls prevention in older persons. 2009. Available at: http://www.medcats.com/FALLS/GOL.htm. Accessed April 10, 2010.

22. Crandall CJ, Newberry SJ, Diamant A, et al. Comparative effectiveness of pharmacologic treatments to prevent fractures: an updated systematic review. Ann Intern Med 2014;161(10):711.

23. Cosman F, et al. Osteoporosis international. London: Springer; 2014. Available at: https://www.ncbi.nlm.nih.gov/pmc/articles/PMC4176573/.

24. Kanis JA, on behalf of the World Health Organization Scientific Group. Assessment of osteoporosis at the primary health-care level. Technical report. United Kingdom: University of Sheffield, WHO Collaborating Centre; 2008. Available

at: https://www.sheffield.ac.uk/FRAX/pdfs/WHO_Technical_Report.pdf. Accessed April 10, 2018.

25. United States Bone and Joint Initiative. The burden of musculoskeletal diseases in the United States (BMUS). 3rd edition. Rosemont (IL): 2014. Available at: http://www.boneandjointburden.org. Accessed April 10, 2010.

26. Becker DJ, Yun H, Kilgore ML, et al. Health services utilization after fractures: evidence from Medicare. J Gerontol A Biol Sci Med Sci 2010;65(9):1012–20.

27. Tajeu GS, Delzell E, Smith W, et al. Death, debility, and destitution following hip fracture. J Gerontol A Biol Sci Med Sci 2014;69(3):346–53.

28. United States Bone and Joint Initiative. The burden of musculoskeletal diseases in the United States (BMUS). 3rd edition. Rosemont (IL): United States Bone and Joint Initiative; 2014. Available at: http://www.boneandjointburden.org. Accessed April 10, 2018.

29. Available at: Uspreventiveservicestaskforce.org. Accessed January 30, 2018.

30. National Osteoporosis Guideline Group (NOGG). Available at: www.sheffield.ac.uk/NOGG/NOGG%20Guideline%202017.pdf. Accessed February 7, 2018.

31. Camacho PM, Petak SM, Binkley N, et al. American Association of Clinical Endocrinologists and American College of Endocrinology clinical practice guidelines for the diagnosis and treatment of postmenopausal osteoporosis - 2016–executive summary. Endocr Pract 2016;22(9):1111–8.

Moving?

Make sure your subscription moves with you!

To notify us of your new address, find your **Clinics Account Number** (located on your mailing label above your name), and contact customer service at:

Email: journalscustomerservice-usa@elsevier.com

800-654-2452 (subscribers in the U.S. & Canada)
314-447-8871 (subscribers outside of the U.S. & Canada)

Fax number: 314-447-8029

Elsevier Health Sciences Division
Subscription Customer Service
3251 Riverport Lane
Maryland Heights, MO 63043

*To ensure uninterrupted delivery of your subscription, please notify us at least 4 weeks in advance of move.

Printed and bound by CPI Group (UK) Ltd, Croydon, CR0 4YY

03/10/2024

01040408-0001